Nursing Care Planning

made

Incredibly Easy!

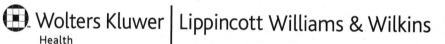

Wolters Kluwer | Lippincott Williams & Wilkins
Health

Philadelphia · Baltimore · New York · London
Buenos Aires · Hong Kong · Sydney · Tokyo

D0702172

RT
41
.N869
2008

·1 13554864

80180117

Staff

+ 1 CD-ROM

Executive Publisher
Judith A. Schilling McCann, RN, MSN

Editorial Director
David Moreau

Clinical Director
Joan M. Robinson, RN, MSN

Art Director
Mary Ludwicki

Electronic Project Manager
John Macalino

Senior Managing Editor
Jaime Stockslager Buss, MSPH, ELS

Clinical Project Manager
Carol A. Saunderson, RN, BA, BS

Editors
Sharon Cole, Karen C. Comerford,
Kathy Goldberg, Sid Karpoff, Diane Labus,
Janeen Levine, Dorothy P. Terry,
Beth Wegerbauer

Clinical Editors
Lisa Morris Bonsall, RN, MSN, CRNP; Nancy
LaPlante, RN, MSN; Anita Lockhart, RNC, MSN;
Kate Stout, RN, MSN, CCRN

Copy Editors
Kimberly Bilotta (supervisor), Scotti Cohn,
Amy Furman, Shana Harrington, Dorothy P. Terry,
Pamela Wingrod

Illustrator
Bot Roda

Designer
Georg W. Purvis IV

Digital Composition Services
Diane Paluba (manager), Joyce Rossi Biletz

Associate Manufacturing Manager
Beth J. Welsh

Editorial Assistants
Karen J. Kirk, Linda K. Ruhf

Indexer
Barbara Hodgson

The clinical treatments described and recommended in this publication are based on research and consultation with nursing, medical, and legal authorities. To the best of our knowledge, these procedures reflect currently accepted practice. Nevertheless, they can't be considered absolute and universal recommendations. For individual applications, all recommendations must be considered in light of the patient's clinical condition and, before administration of new or infrequently used drugs, in light of the latest package-insert information. The authors and publisher disclaim any responsibility for any adverse effects resulting from the suggested procedures, from any undetected errors, or from the reader's misunderstanding of the text.

© 2008 by Lippincott Williams & Wilkins. All rights reserved. This book is protected by copyright. No part of it may be reproduced, stored in a retrieval system, or transmitted, in any form or by any means—electronic, mechanical, photocopy, recording, or otherwise—without prior written permission of the publisher, except for brief quotations embodied in critical articles and reviews and testing and evaluation materials provided by publisher to instructors whose schools have adopted its accompanying textbook. Printed in the United States of America. For information, write Lippincott Williams & Wilkins, 323 Norristown Road, Suite 200, Ambler, PA 19002-2756.

NCPIE010407

Library of Congress Cataloging-in-Publication Data
Nursing care planning made incredibly easy.
    p. ; cm.
    Includes bibliographical references and index.
    1. Nursing care plans—Handbooks, manuals, etc. 2. Nursing—Planning—Handbooks, manuals, etc. 3. Nursing diagnosis—Handbooks, manuals, etc. I. Lippincott Williams & Wilkins.
    [DNLM: 1. Nursing Process—Examination Questions. 2. Nursing Process—Handbooks. 3. Patient Care Planning—Examination Questions. 4.
    Patient Care Planning—Handbooks. WY 49 N974295 2007]
RT41.N8778 2007
610.73—dc22
ISBN-13: 978-1-58255-553-9 (alk. paper)
ISBN-10: 1-58255-553-2 (alk. paper)   2007001378

Contents

Advisory board   *iv*

Contributors and consultants   *v*

Foreword   *vii*

Part I   Care planning using the nursing process

1	Introduction to care planning	3
2	Assessment	23
3	Nursing diagnosis	61
4	Planning	87
5	Implementation	119
6	Evaluation	143
7	Putting it all together	159

Part II   Nursing diagnoses by medical diagnosis

8	Medical-surgical diagnoses	191
9	Maternal-neonatal diagnoses	245
10	Pediatric diagnoses	251
11	Psychiatric diagnoses	263

Appendices and index

NANDA-I nursing diagnoses by domain   *272*

Selected references   *274*

Index   *275*

Advisory board

Ivy Alexander, PhD, CANP
Assistant Professor
Yale University
New Haven, Conn.

Susan E. Appling, RN, MS, CRNP
Assistant Professor
Johns Hopkins University School of Nursing
Baltimore

Paul M. Arnstein, PhD, APRN-BC, FNP-C
Assistant Professor
Boston College
Boston

Bobbie Berkowitz, PhD, CNAA, FAAN
Chair & Professor
Psychosocial & Community Health
University of Washington
Seattle

Karla Jones, RN, MSN
Nursing Faculty
Treasure Valley Community College
Ontario, Ore.

Manon Lemonde, PhD, RN
Associate Professor
University of Ontario Institute of Technology
Oshawa, Ontario, Canada

Sheila Sparks Ralph, DNSC, RN, FAAN
Director & Professor, Division of Nursing & Respiratory Care
Shenandoah University
Winchester, Va.

Kristine Anne Scordo, PhD, RN, CS, ACNP
Director, Acute Care Nurse Practitioner Program
Wright State University
Dayton, Ohio

Robin Wilkerson, PhD, RN,BC
Associate Professor
University of Mississippi
Jackson

Contributors and consultants

Melody C. Antoon, RN, MSN
Instructor
Lamar State College
Port Arthur, Tex.

Elizabeth (Libby) A. Archer, RN, EDD
Associate Professor
Baptist College of Health Sciences
Memphis

Peggy D. Baikie, RNC, MS, NNP, PNP
Clinical Coordinator/Nurse Practitioner
St. Anthony Hospitals
Denver
Adjunct Professor
Metropolitan State College of Denver

Mary Elaine Bell-Braxton, RN, MS
Adjunct Faculty & Nursing Resource Center Coordinator
University of West Georgia
Carrollton

Cheryl L. Brady, RN, MSN
Assistant Professor
Kent State University
Salem, Ohio

Stephanie C. Butkus, RN, MSN, CPNP, IBCLC
Assistant Professor, Division of Nursing
Kettering (Ohio) College of Medical Arts

Joanna E. Cain, RN, BSN
President
Auctorial Pursuits, Inc.
Wilmington, N.C.

Julie Calvery, RN, MS
Instructor
University of Arkansas
Fort Smith

Cynthia A. Chatham, RNC, DSN
Associate Professor
University of Southern Mississippi School of Nursing
Long Beach

Wendy Tagan Conroy, MSN, FNP,BC
Advanced Practice Registered Nurse
Connecticut Valley Hospital
Middletown

Charlotte Conway, RN, MSN
Per Diem Staff Nurse, Pediatric Intensive Care
Santa Clara Valley Medical Center
San Jose, Calif.

Linda Carman Copel, RN, PhD, CGP, CS, DAPA
Associate Professor
Villanova (Pa.) University

Linda Crawford, RN, MSN
Assistant Professor of Practical Nursing
Coastal Georgia Community College
Brunswick

Kim R. Davis, RN, MSN
Nurse Manager, MICU and SICU
Ralph H. Johnson VA Medical Center
Charleston, S.C.

Valerie J. Flattes, APRN, BC-ANP
Clinical Instructor
University of Utah College of Nursing
Salt Lake City

Erica Fooshee, RN, MSN
Nursing Instructor
Department of Nursing
Pensacola (Fla.) Junior College

Candace Furlong, APRN,BC, MSN, CNS, NP
Professor, Nursing
American River College
Sacramento, Calif.

Rhonda Gall, APRN,BC, GNP
Lecturer
Bowie (Md.) State University

Janis Guilbeau, RN, MSN
Instructor of Nursing
University of Louisiana
Lafayette

Kenneth Hazell, ARNP, MSN, PhD(c)
Nursing Program Director
Keiser University
Ft. Lauderdale, Fla.

Connie S. Heflin, RN, MSN
Professor
West Kentucky Community and Technical College
Paducah

Julia Anne Isen, RN, MS, FNP-C
Assistant Clinical Professor,
    School of Nursing
University of California
San Francisco

Karla Jones, RN, MN
Nursing Department Faculty
Treasure Valley Community
    College
Ontario, Ore.

Rebecca Frey Keller, ARNP, MSN
Nursing Instructor
Keiser College
Fort Lauderdale, Fla.

Merita Konstantacos, RN, MSN
Consultant
Clinton, Ohio

Cheryl Laskowski, APRN-BC, DNS
Assistant Professor of Nursing
University of Vermont
Burlington
Advanced Practice Nurse
Center for Pain Medicine
South Burlington, Vt.

Rosemary Macy, RN, PhD
Associate Professor
Boise (Idaho) State University

Judith A. Murphy, RN, BSN
Ambulatory Nurse
Cambridge Health Alliance
Medford, Mass.

Noel C. Piano, RN, MS
Instructor/Coordinator
Lafayette School of Practical
    Nursing
Adjunct Faculty
Thomas Nelson Community
    College
Williamsburg, Va.

Melody F. Pope, RN, MSED, MSN
Assistant Professor of Nursing
College of the Redwoods
Crescent City, Calif.

Monica Narvaez Ramirez, RN,
    MSN
Nursing Instructor
University of the Incarnate Word
    School of Nursing & Health
    Professions
San Antonio, Tex.

Debra L. Renna, CCRN, MSN
Professor of Nursing
Keiser College
Fort Lauderdale, Fla.

Nan C. Riedè, RN, MSN
Assistant Professor
Baptist College of Health
    Sciences
Memphis

Barbara K. Scheirer, RN, MSN
Assistant Professor
School of Nursing
Grambling (La.) State University

Kendra S. Seiler, RN, MSN
Nursing Instructor
Rio Hondo College
Whittier, Calif.

Georgia Simmons, RN, BSN
Practical Nursing Instructor
Ivy Tech Community College
Madison, Ind.

Sheryl Thomas, RN, MSN
Nurse Instructor
Wayne County Community
    College
Detroit

Phyllis Tipton, RN, PhD
ADN Instructor
McLennan Community College
Research Coordinator
Hillcrest Baptist Medical Center
Waco, Tex.

Kathleen Tusaie, APRN, BC, PhD
Assistant Professor/Advanced
    Practice Nurse
The University of Akron (Ohio)
    College of Nursing

Patricia Van Tine, RN, MA, CPT
Nursing Educator
Mt. San Jacinto College
Menifee, Calif.

Ralph Vogel, RN, PhD, CPNP
Assistant Clinical Professor
College of Nursing
University of Arkansas for
    Medical Sciences
Little Rock

Sandra K. Voll, RNC, MS, CNM, FNP,
    WHNP
Clinical Assistant Professor,
    Director of Clinical Learning
    Center
Virginia Commonwealth Universi-
    ty School of Nursing
Richmond

Kelly Witter, RN, MSN, CLC
Director, Practical Nursing
    Program
Great Oaks Career Campuses
Cincinnati

Hollace Yowler, RN, MSN
Associate Professor
Ivy Tech Community College
Madison, Ind.

Foreword

I am a nursing process believer! Throughout my academic and practice careers, I have consistently used the nursing process to help me, and my students, make sense of patients' clinical presentation, pathophysiology, treatments, and nursing care. I also believe that there's a little private eye or puzzle solver in each nurse. Trying to make sense of assessment data, laboratory findings, responses to care provided, and other data requires critical thinking and problem-solving skills. However, these tasks also keep the practice of nursing fresh, exciting, and challenging! One tool for making these tasks less demanding is the nursing process; and one extraordinary resource for making the nursing process less unwieldy is *Nursing Care Planning Made Incredibly Easy.*

The nursing process is the foundation for professional nursing practice. It's the systematic, problem-solving method used to teach and guide nursing care planning. Practicing nurses use the nursing process as the framework for the clinical decision making and critical thinking that are essential for safe, quality nursing practice. In addition, clinical guidelines, care maps, and standards of care are all based on the nursing process. Students develop care plans in nursing school to learn the nursing process and to learn how to implement it in practice.

Nursing Care Planning Made Incredibly Easy takes an innovative approach to nursing care planning in that it focuses on the skills necessary to develop patient-specific, relevant, timely nursing care plans. Divided into two sections, this unique new reference walks students step-by-step through the care planning process in a way that builds problem-solving and critical-thinking skills. Content that's particularly valuable to nursing students includes discussions about the differences between medical and nursing diagnoses; the relevance of nursing care planning to practice after graduation; techniques for developing a practical care plan the day before clinical; NANDA International (NANDA-I), NIC, and NOC and ways in which these classification systems can be used together; the role of the nurse and nursing documentation in interdisciplinary care; and the importance of evaluation throughout patient care. The importance of systematic problem solving is emphasized throughout the text through the use of concept maps, sample case studies, and sample care plan components. Important terms are defined and applied to aid student comprehension of these important concepts.

Part I of the book is dedicated to the development of a nursing care plan and details each step of the nursing process. Following the five-step nursing process—assessment, diagnosis, planning, implementation, and evaluation—each chapter includes a detailed discussion of the step and its application to nursing practice, with loads of practical application examples. Each chapter ends with *On the case*, a quiz that helps students hone their critical-thinking skills and gauge their comprehension of the content presented. Part II, "Nursing diagnoses by medical diagnosis," is a handy resource that lists hundreds of examples of medical-surgical, psychiatric, maternal-neonatal, and pediatric nursing diagnoses for the most common medical diagnoses. The book also includes a free CD-ROM with more than 150 customizable care plans from every nursing specialty.

Logos throughout the text make learning easy and focus the reader on essential information:

Under construction offers sample concept maps and care plan components, plus tips for making care plans patient specific and individualized

Weighing the evidence provides information on the latest evidenced-based standards of care used in the sample care plans

Teacher knows best imparts important reminders from Instructor Joy that help students understand how to apply content

Memory jogger mnemonic devices help students remember key concepts and content.

In summary, *Nursing Care Planning Made Incredibly Easy* is a valuable reference for nursing students learning the nursing process and nursing care planning. I believe this text will not only assist the student in learning how to develop an individualized care plan but, more importantly, it will provide a framework for using the nursing process to better understand the clinical presentation and nursing care needs of the patient as well as to promote systematic problem-solving and clinical judgment.

Janice J. Hoffman, RN, PhD
Faculty
Johns-Hopkins University School of Nursing
Baltimore

Part I Care planning using the nursing process

1 Introduction to care planning   3

2 Assessment   23

3 Nursing diagnosis   61

4 Planning   87

5 Implementation   119

6 Evaluation   143

7 Putting it all together   159

Introduction to care planning

Just the facts

In this chapter, you'll learn:

♦ the benefits of using the nursing process

♦ the role of the nursing process in planning patient care

♦ ways in which the nursing process promotes critical thinking

♦ fundamentals of concept mapping and its uses in care planning.

A look at care planning

A crucial component of nursing care, a care plan (also known as a *plan of care*) serves as a road map that guides all staff members involved in a patient's care. Care planning allows a nurse to identify a patient's problems and select interventions that will help solve or minimize these problems.

The great communicator

The care plan also communicates vital patient information to the entire health care team. It contains detailed instructions for achieving the goals established for the patient.

Think of a care plan as a map that helps the health care team stay on course when it comes to patient care.

Understanding the nursing process

Effective care planning results from the nursing process—a deliberate, systematic process that takes a problem-solving approach to nursing care. Development and acceptance of the nursing process is one of the key advances in nursing over the past few decades.

Analyze, address, implement, evaluate

The cornerstone of clinical nursing, the nursing process gives you a structure for applying your knowledge and skills in an organized, goal-oriented way. It helps you think critically, solve problems, and make care decisions tailored to each patient's individual needs.

The nursing process requires you to systematically analyze patient data, make inferences, draw conclusions about patient problems, devise a care plan to address those problems, implement the plan, evaluate the plan's effectiveness, and revise the plan if necessary.

Oh, the humanity

The nursing process is holistic and humanistic. It addresses the human response to medical conditions—how these conditions affect the patient's life. To use it correctly, you must consider not just the patient's physical, mental, and emotional status but also his interests, values, beliefs, and ethnic, religious, and cultural background.

Advantages of the nursing process

When used effectively, the nursing process offers many advantages:
- It's patient centered, helping to ensure that your patient's health problems and his response to them are the focus of care.
- It enables you to individualize care for each patient.
- It promotes the patient's participation in his care, encourages independence and compliance, and gives the patient a greater sense of control—important factors in a positive health outcome. (See *Putting the "P" in planning*.)

Teacher knows best

Putting the "P" in planning

Always remember to include the "P"—the patient—in planning. Ask for your patient's input when identifying his problems, establishing outcomes, and formulating interventions. Doing this validates his importance as an individual and motivates him to participate in his health care and adhere to the care plan. It also gives him a greater sense of control, which promotes personal responsibility and strengthens his commitment to working toward the established goals.

• It improves communication by providing you and other nurses with a common list of the patient's recognized health problems.
• It promotes accountability for nursing activities based on evaluation, which in turn promotes quality assurance.
• It promotes critical thinking, decision making, and problem solving.
• It's outcome-focused and encourages the evaluation of results.
• It minimizes errors and omissions in care planning.

Basis for the nursing process

The nursing process is based on the scientific method of problem solving, which involves:
• stating the problem you observed
• forming a hypothesis about the solution to the problem ("if…then" statements)
• developing a method to test the hypothesis
• collecting the test data
• analyzing the data
• drawing conclusions about the hypothesis.

A scientific fact

Most people use the scientific method instinctively, without being aware they're doing it. Simply picking out which pair of shoes best complements your favorite outfit is an exercise in the scientific method. So if you're familiar with the scientific process, the nursing process probably seems familiar.

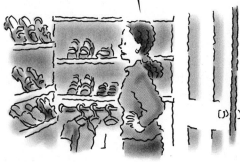

Picking out shoes is scientific? I knew there was a good reason it took me so long—I just always thought it was all of the shoes.

Nursing process steps

The nursing process encompasses five steps:

assessment

nursing diagnosis

planning

implementation

evaluation.

Following these steps systematically in this order enables you to organize and prioritize patient care—especially critical for the novice nursing student. It also helps ensure that you don't skip or overlook important information. (See *Just how many steps are there?*, page 6.)

Just how many steps are there?

Nurses are accountable for maintaining national practice standards, such as those set by the American Nurses Association (ANA). These standards state that "...the nursing process encompasses all significant actions taken by registered nurses and forms the foundation for decision-making." However, the number of nursing process steps into which this definition translates varies.

The initial definition of the nursing process from the 1950s listed only three steps: assessment, planning, and evaluation. However, the ANA cites six steps in the nursing process:
• assessment
• nursing diagnosis
• outcome identification
• planning
• implementation
• evaluation.
Many authors and instructors have found it useful to combine outcome identification into the planning step because it's so closely allied to the choice of appropriate nursing interventions.

Remember that the nursing process guides all the nurse's *actions* and *decisions,* regardless of the number of steps cited.

When used correctly, the nursing process ensures that the care plan is revised when new problems arise or patient outcomes remain unmet. It also allows the care plan to be discontinued when patient outcomes have been met.

Domino effect

Although the five nursing process steps are sequential, they also are continuous and overlapping. For instance, when performing an intervention, such as changing your patient's dressing, you should also be assessing his skin. (See *The nursing process: An unbroken circle.*)

What's more, these steps are interrelated, with each one influencing all the subsequent steps. For instance:
• Your assessment must be thorough and accurate so that you formulate the appropriate nursing diagnosis.
• The nursing diagnosis you formulate must be appropriate to ensure that you choose reasonable outcomes.
• The outcomes you identify must be appropriate so that you outline correct interventions.
• The interventions you choose must be appropriate so that your patient will make progress toward the outcomes you've established.

The nursing process: An unbroken circle

The nursing process is a progression of actions that continually recycle as patient problems and priorities change or resolve. In any specific task you do, more than one step may be involved.

Take for example...

When you initially assess a new patient's lungs, you begin the process of determining if the patient has any actual or potential problems related to respiratory function. In addition to assessing respiratory function, you can assess the skin integrity on the patient's chest and back.

The next time you assess his lungs, you can evaluate whether an intervention teaching him to use an incentive spirometer was effective in keeping his lungs clear. When you do this, however, you notice that his apical heart beat is rapid and irregular—a change from your initial *assessment.* Now you quickly:

• conclude that the spirometry has been effective so far (*evaluation*)

• identify that the patient is at risk for decreased cardiac output (*nursing diagnosis*)

• identify that the patient's heart rate should return to less than 100 beats/minute with a regular rhythm (*planning expected outcomes*)

• determine that you should ask the patient how he's feeling to identify associated symptoms, check the patient's pulse oximetry to assess the need for supportive oxygen, obtain an immediate 12-lead electrocardiogram, and notify the practitioner of the change (*planning interventions*)

• put your devised plan into action (*implementation*).

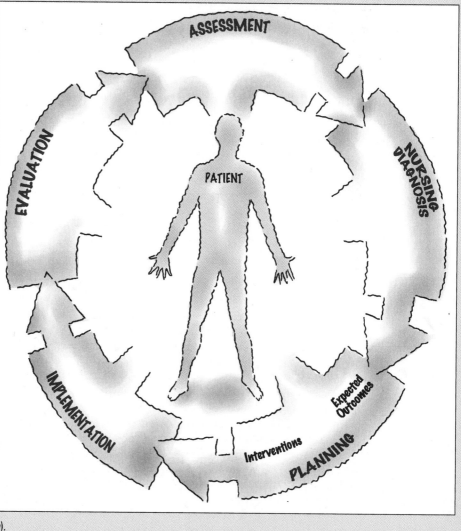

Under construction

Actual vs. *Risk for* nursing diagnoses

When formulating your patient's nursing diagnoses, you need to specify whether your patient has each problem or is at risk for developing it. Here's the distinction:

• If the patient has identifiable signs and symptoms that appear in all or most patients with the disorder, you should label the problem with an *actual* nursing diagnosis.

• If the patient has risk factors for a problem but doesn't have signs or symptoms, you should label the problem with a *Risk for* diagnosis.

Take impaired skin integrity, for example. If the patient has erythema or an open skin area, he has *actual* impaired skin integrity and his diagnosis would be *Impaired skin integrity*. If he has no signs of skin breakdown but is bedbound and has bowel and bladder incontinence, he has predisposing factors that place him at risk for impaired skin integrity; therefore, his nursing diagnosis would be *Risk for impaired skin integrity*.

If you go astray during any step—say, by misinterpreting the assessment data—you can get back on track by reassessing the patient, evaluating his care plan, and revising the plan if necessary.

Assessment

The first step in the nursing process, assessment involves the systematic collection of patient data. A comprehensive assessment gives you a wide-angle view of your patient's health problems, aiding in crucial decisions about patient care.

Nursing diagnosis

The second step requires you to use your assessment data to formulate nursing diagnoses—clinical judgments about the patient's response to an actual or potential health problem that nurses are legally permitted to manage. (See *Actual vs.* Risk for *diagnoses.*) Remember, nursing diagnoses are different from medical diagnoses. (See *How nursing and medical diagnoses differ.*)

After the patient's problems or responses have been identified and reframed as nursing diagnoses, a quick review of the assessment findings and diagnoses can help you to correctly prioritize the most urgent needs of the patient.

> Although both are important parts of patient care, medical and nursing diagnoses are different.

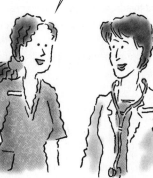

How nursing and medical diagnoses differ

Practitioners such as doctors, nurse practitioners, and physician assistants diagnose and treat medical conditions related to anatomy, physiology, disease, or trauma. They formulate medical diagnoses that center on these medical diseases and conditions.

Nurses aren't licensed to diagnose medical diseases and conditions. Instead, they formulate nursing diagnoses that focus on how the patient responds to the medical disease or condition. Unlike medical diagnoses, nursing diagnoses are patient-centered.

This case study will help you understand the difference between medical and nursing diagnoses.

Point, counterpoint
Mr. Mills is a 52-year-old man who was hospitalized after falling on a patch of ice and injuring his right hip. He's married and has two children, one of whom attends college. Mr. Mills works as a construction foreman; his wife is unemployed.

The practitioner's viewpoint
Here's how the practitioner sees the situation: Mr. Mills presents with pain in the right hip, a shortened right leg, and external rotation of the right hip after sustaining a fall on a patch of ice. The hip X-ray shows a well-defined intertrochanteric fracture of the right hip. The medical diagnosis is a *right hip fracture*. The medical plan is to proceed with open reduction and internal fixation of the hip.

The nurse's perspective
Here's how the nurse views the same patient information: Mr. Mills has pain in his right hip. He expresses an immediate concern about the need to urinate. He's also concerned about his job and lack of income during the recuperation period, when he won't be able to work. He says he has always been the breadwinner of his family, and he's worried that if he needs to be off work for a long time, he won't have the money to pay his son's college tuition. The initial nursing diagnoses for Mr. Mills are *Acute pain related to right hip fracture; Impaired urinary elimination related to inability to stand, pain, and voluntary retention; Anxiety related to financial concerns; and Risk for situational low self-esteem related to anticipated loss of roles as employee and family provider.*

The differences
The nurse focuses on Mr. Mills and his *responses* to the hip fracture. She isn't licensed to treat the patient's hip fracture independently but can address problems stemming from his responses to the fracture, such as pain and discomfort, concern with urination, and the expected role change.

The nursing care plan should address Mr. Mills' pain management needs, should include education about the indwelling urinary catheter that the nurse will place, a social service consult to address Mr. Mills' financial concerns, and assistance in working through his expected role changes.

Three's company

Each nursing diagnosis has three components:
* label—an actual or potential problem that nursing care can affect

• related factors—factors that may precede, contribute to, or be associated with the human response
• evidence—signs and symptoms that point to the nursing diagnosis.

Suppose, for instance, that your patient has constipation resulting from use of opioid analgesics for pain. You would formulate a nursing diagnosis of *Constipation related to use of opioid analgesics as evidenced by passage of hard, formed stools.*

One thing leads to another

Correctly identifying the problem and its cause is crucial to the next steps of the nursing process—planning and implementation.

Planning

During the planning stage of the nursing process, you:
• identify expected patient outcomes, or goals
• select nursing interventions designed to achieve these outcomes
• document the care plan, which becomes a permanent part of the patient's record and communicates the patient's needs to all health care providers who use the plan.

Here come the outcomes

For every nursing diagnosis, you must identify expected outcomes—measurable, patient-focused, time-specific goals the patient should reach as a result of the nursing interventions you've planned.

Outcomes derive from the nursing diagnosis. You must state them in terms of the patient's behavior. For example, if the patient has a nursing diagnosis of *Deficient knowledge (incision care)*, one reasonable outcome might be "Patient will verbalize precautions to take to prevent incision infection until healed."

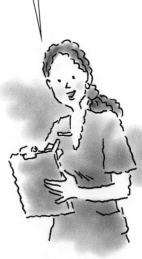

Don't forget documentation. It's an important part of the process.

Next in line—the interventions

Once you've identified the patient's problem or response and determined a reasonable outcome measurement, you can begin to list the steps that must be taken to reach that goal. Interventions are brief descriptions of specific actions. They should be based on the best evidence available documenting effectiveness and validity for achieving the desired outcome, and they should conform to appropriate standards of care.

Don't forget to document

Always document the care plan so it's accessible to other staff members. Doing this provides crucial patient information to other health care team members, promoting continuity of care.

Implementation

The next step in the nursing process is implementation, when you perform the actual interventions to help your patient reach the expected outcomes. But before carrying out these interventions, be sure to quickly reassess the patient to make sure that the interventions you've planned are still necessary. Patient situations can change rapidly, making some interventions inappropriate or unnecessary.

Throughout your nursing care, you'll need to evaluate the effectiveness of your interventions and make changes as needed. If you continue to implement ineffective interventions, you and your patient will lose valuable time. (See *Be pliable about care plans*.)

Evaluation

During the evaluation step of the nursing process, you:
• reassess the patient
• compare your findings with the outcome criteria you established during the planning step
• determine the extent of outcome achievement—whether the outcome was fully met, partially met, or not met at all
• write evaluation statements
• revise the care plan as needed.

Although technically the last step of the nursing process, evaluation is an ongoing process that occurs each time you see the patient. You must continually evaluate the patient's response to interventions. (See *The focus factor*, page 12.)

A change of plans

If desired outcomes have been achieved, the care plan may be discontinued. If an outcome has been partially met, the plan may be continued with an extended time line.

If a desired outcome hasn't been met, you must reexamine the care plan and make necessary changes. To change the plan, you may need to review the new assessment data, formulate new diagnoses, establish new outcomes, and select new interventions. Then update the written care plan accordingly.

How the nursing process promotes critical thinking

To use the nursing process, you must be able to think critically. Critical thinking is a disciplined mental process of analyzing problems or phenomena that have been gathered from observation, experience, reflection, reasoning, or communication.

Deliberate, purposeful, and conscious, critical thinking requires reasonable, rational interpretation and evaluation of infor-

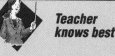

Teacher knows best

Be pliable about care plans

The nursing care plan isn't set in stone. It must be updated as your patient's problems, needs, and priorities change. Be sure to review the care plan often and modify it when necessary.

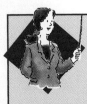

The focus factor

Stay focused during all interactions with your patient. To do this, you'll need to use active listening skills and turn off other thoughts going through your head, including "What should I make for dinner?" and "What time is my dentist appointment tomorrow?" Most patients are aware of the amount of focus and interest you bring to an exchange and will respond in kind.

mation. It leads you to reasonable solutions to a problem and helps you choose among these possible solutions to make a decision.

Hallmarks of critical thinking

The hallmarks of critical thinking are:
• clear, careful, and precise thinking
• objective analysis of the evidence
• use of logical reasoning to reach a discriminating decision
• elimination of stereotypical thinking, bias, preconceptions, and emotionally charged thinking.

A model process

The nursing process is a model of critical thinking because each step is purposeful, deliberate, and designed to attain a certain goal. (See *Critical thinking: An essential skill.*)

For instance, when evaluating the assessment data you've gathered, you must think critically to determine which questions to ask your patient next. If he says he occasionally experiences chest pain, the critically thinking nurse doesn't simply record this statement and move on to the next topic. Instead, she asks questions designed to elicit details about the chest pain, such as:
• When does the pain occur? Do you experience it after strenuous physical activity? Does it occur after meals? While resting?
• How severe is the pain on a scale of 0 to 10?
• Do you have other problems along with the pain?
• Does the pain radiate to other parts of your body?

Risky factors

Thinking critically during assessment enables you to recognize factors that place your patient at increased risk for developing a problem. If you detect such a potential, you'll know the care plan should include a *Risk for* nursing diagnosis and appropriate interventions to prevent the problem.

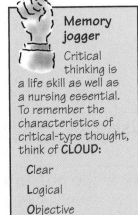

Memory jogger

Critical thinking is a life skill as well as a nursing essential. To remember the characteristics of critical-type thought, think of **CLOUD:**

Clear

Logical

Objective

Unbiased

Dispassionate (not emotion-driven).

Critical thinking: An essential skill

In the complex, rapidly changing health care environment, safe and effective nursing care demands critical thinking. Taking basic problem solving one step further, critical thinking considers all related factors, including the patient's unique needs and individual differences. Critical-thinking skills allow the nurse to step outside the situation and look at the whole picture more objectively.

Truth seekers

To obtain this complete picture, critical thinkers seek the truth and actively pursue answers to questions. They're also open-minded and creative and can draw from past clinical experience to come up with all possible alternatives and then zero in on the best solution for the patient.

Practice for your practice

Books, articles, and online courses are available to hone nurses' critical-thinking skills. When nurses engage in critical thinking, their patients have the best chances for success.

Likewise, critical thinking helps you write outcomes in a way that promotes easier evaluation and makes the need for any revisions readily apparent.

Novices need it, too

Critical thinking skills are essential for nurses at every level. As a novice nurse, you'll encounter situations you didn't see or learn about during your student clinical rotation—complex problems that require sound decision-making skills. You'll be expected to make important patient-care decisions and take actions based on those decisions.

As technology grows more advanced, such decisions and actions are becoming increasingly complex. What's more, they require you to analyze many patient variables, including social, cultural, emotional, physical, financial, and spiritual issues.

Using the nursing process after graduation

No matter how thoroughly you're oriented in your first nursing job, you'll confront many new and unfamiliar situations throughout your career. You'll need to make many on-the-spot decisions—some of which will be crucial. Using the nursing process and critical thinking skills will help you succeed no matter what your responsibilities are. As you become more familiar with the nursing process, gain experience writing care plans, and hone your critical-thinking skills, your clinical judgment and ability to make good decisions undoubtedly will improve.

Roll with the changes

Because the patient's status is dynamic and can change quickly, the nursing process is dynamic as well. As your patient's condition changes, you must assess these changes quickly and adjust the care plan appropriately. Use the nursing process as a road map and critical thinking as the vehicle to take you and your patient to the destination—the desired patient outcome.

Rinse and repeat

As you gain experience, you'll see that the nursing process shows you when and how to stop a nursing intervention—namely, when the desired outcomes are met. Or, if the outcomes remain unmet, the nursing process will lead you to reassess the situation and, if necessary, repeat the entire process.

Understanding NANDA-I, NOC, and NIC

Using standard terminology in the care plan helps ensure that all members of the nursing team have the same understanding of the patient's needs. Technology and the increasing use of electronic medical records have increased the need for standardized nursing language.

Speaking the same language

Several standardized classification systems exist for nursing diagnoses, outcomes, and interventions. With these systems, you can use a single term to describe what otherwise would require several words.

NANDA-I diagnoses

Most nurses use the diagnoses identified by NANDA International (NANDA-I; formerly the North American Nursing Diagnosis Association). NANDA-I develops standardized nursing diagnosis terminology for nurses at all levels and in all practice areas.

NANDA-I was founded in 1973 during a conference held to establish a classification system for nursing diagnoses. In 1987, the American Nurses Association authorized NANDA-I as the governing organization for development of a nursing diagnosis classification system. NANDA-I meets periodically to review and accept new diagnoses or, when necessary, to revise previously accepted diagnoses. It then publishes the updated, revised list of approved diagnoses.

Other classification systems

The Nursing Outcomes Classification (NOC) system, developed at the University of Iowa School of Nursing, is a standardized classification system for patient outcomes that helps nurses evaluate the effects of nursing interventions.

NOC is no laughing matter

NOC outcomes can be used in all settings across the care continuum to follow patient outcomes throughout an illness episode or over an extended time. The NOC system consists of 330 outcomes organized into 29 classes and 7 domains. Each outcome has a definition and a list of measurable indicators. (See *Don't knock NOC!*)

NIC follows NOC

The Nursing Interventions Classification (NIC) is a comprehensive, research-based standardized classification system for interventions that nurses perform. Like the NOC system, it was developed at the University of Iowa School of Nursing. NIC addresses both the physiologic and psychosocial aspects of nursing care and includes independent and collaborative interventions.

Research conducted and used in formulating NIC helps ensure that nursing interventions are based on the best evidence—not guesswork. Evidence-based interventions promote the best patient outcomes and take the guesswork out of planning care. (See *NIC and nurses*, page 16.)

Weighing the evidence

Don't knock NOC!

Classification of nursing outcomes was initiated in the 1970s in response to a need to identify and measure outcomes of patient care that were responsive to nursing practices. To establish appropriate reimbursement and determine reasonable staffing coverage, health care organizations, insurers, and regulators wanted to measure how the nursing care provided affected the patient's health status. Nurses themselves wanted a language that demonstrated the uniqueness of their profession and provided a framework for further nursing research.

The nursing outcomes listed by the Iowa Outcomes Project 2004 Nursing Outcomes Classification (NOC) are research based and have been evaluated for reliability, validity, and sensitivity. Therefore, NOC outcomes provide an excellent guideline in the preparation of standardized or individualized care plans, paving the way for evidence-based nursing practice.

Weighing the evidence

NIC and nurses

Research for a classification of nursing interventions began in 1987. Nurses needed a clear, concise, and measurable list of nursing actions to ease documentation time, aid interdisciplinary communication, assess productivity and competency, foster nursing research, and teach nursing students. These nursing actions were grouped together into broader categories of interventions specific to particular patient outcomes.

For example, the *intervention* "Cardiac Care" contains a list of specific *nursing activities* that partially includes evaluation of chest pain, assessment of peripheral circulation, documentation of cardiac arrhythmia, and promotion of stress reduction. The specific nursing activities listed are based on research and standards of care from relevant professional organizations, and each intervention includes a definition and selected references.

The interventions listed on an individual care plan are ultimately based on the clinical judgment of the nurse responsible for the patient's care. Nursing activities cited must be modified to reflect unique actions required to help that patient meet his desired outcomes. Actions that don't apply to the patient should be omitted. This feature of NIC is what guarantees that nurses remain patient focused and in control of the nursing process.

Language link-ups

Over the past several years, members of the research teams responsible for NANDA, NIC, and NOC have consulted to develop linkages (terminology that links one classification system to the others). Together, the three classifications provide the basics for a complete care plan. This gives all nurses a common understanding of nursing care.

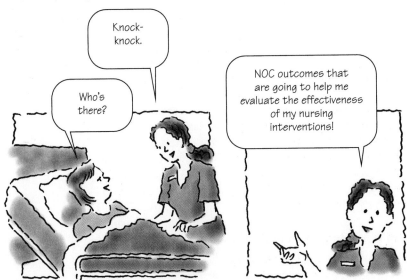

Concept mapping

A common tool to assist you in critical thinking is a concept map (sometimes called a *mind map*). A concept map is a diagram that shows relationships among various concepts. Concept mapping is a tool for visualizing how concepts relate to one another. It helps you understand your patient's problems and care needs—and see how these items interact with each other.

A concept map helps you organize your thinking and see the big clinical picture. Each concept is enclosed in a box or circle, with lines between related concepts. Concept maps are especially helpful if you're a visual learner.

Comparing concept mapping and care planning

Concept mapping and traditional nursing care planning both have a problem-solving focus. However, concept mapping doesn't require linear design, which can hinder the free flow of ideas. It lets you view information in different ways and from different viewpoints because concepts aren't locked into specific positions. (See *Quick comparison*, page 18.)

Advantages of concept mapping

Concept mapping also has these other advantages over the traditional care plan:
• It makes the seemingly intangible concepts of patient problems, causes, and effects more manageable.
• It clearly defines the central concept (the patient problem) by positioning it in the center of the page. This ensures that the patient—not the medical diagnosis—is the focus.
• It shows the relative importance of each concept.
• It helps you identify relationships between important concepts.
• It requires much less time to write than a care plan.
• It encourages creative and innovative ideas.
• It provides all the basic information on one page.
• It allows new information to be easily added.
• It enables you to see contradictions and gaps in the material or its interpretation, which provides a foundation for questioning, discovery, and creativity.

Disadvantages of concept mapping

Despite its advantages, concept mapping can have certain drawbacks:

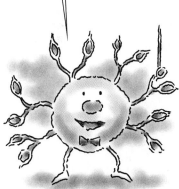

Concept mapping is similar to the brain's neural network. Each concept has long fibers that reach out and connect to other concepts.

Quick comparison

Here's a quick comparison of concept mapping and nursing care plans.

Concept map	Nursing care plan
• Visually organized	• Linearly organized
• Assessment data clearly linked to nursing problems (diagnoses)	• Assessment data usually in separate area or different form
• Good for quick identification and outline of multiple patient problems	• Good for quick communication of priority problems, outcomes, and interventions

• Getting the map just right can be time consuming. You may have to redraw it several times until you're satisfied.
• It may become complex and cluttered, hindering your ability to see the big picture.
• It doesn't easily lend itself to standardized formats for everyday use in the clinical setting.

Creating a concept map

To develop a concept map for your patient, start with a clean sheet of unlined paper. (If you must use lined paper, turn it so the lines are vertical.) To promote creative thinking, you may want to use colored pencils or pens. Then follow these steps:
• After you've assessed your patient, place a circle representing the patient in the middle of the paper. In this circle, write the patient's name or initials, chief complaint, and medical diagnosis. (See example at left.) By placing the patient in the center of the page, your focus is clearly patient centered. Remember, be brief!
• Write the patient's major problems or nursing diagnoses in boxes surrounding the patient, along with pertinent supporting data.
• Use lines to connect the central circle—the patient—to the nursing diagnoses boxes. You may also draw lines between related nursing diagnoses. For example, for a postoperative patient experiencing constipation caused by use of opioid analgesics, you would draw a line between the nursing diagnoses of *Acute pain* and *Constipation* to show that you understand they're related. (See example at right.)
• Write expected outcomes for each nursing diagnosis; place each outcome in its own box because corresponding interventions will

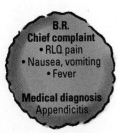

B.R.
Chief complaint
• RLQ pain
• Nausea, vomiting
• Fever

Medical diagnosis
Appendicitis

Acute pain
• Verbalized incisional pain
• Rates pain as 9 on pain scale

B.R.
Chief complaint
• RLQ pain
• Nausea, vomiting
• Fever

Medical diagnosis
Appendicitis

Constipation
• Distended abdomen
• Inability to pass stool

differ for each outcome. Connect these boxes with lines to the appropriate nursing diagnosis.
• In the same way, write interventions in a box for each outcome, followed by evaluations. Draw lines between each part of the nursing process to link related concepts. (See *Concept mapping without tears.*)

Patterns, symbols, and notes

To help clarify your concept map, try using patterns and symbols to help organize types of information, such as:
• branches, to show how a concept can branches into ideas that are either closely or distantly related
• arrows, to join ideas from different branches
• circled groupings, to combine several branches of related ideas.
   You may also include explanatory notes—such as a few words, phrases, or sentences—to explain, question, or comment on a particular point.

Using your concept map

Concept maps are such useful tools that they can be used for multiple purposes. For example, you can use a concept map to analyze a case study for class or to guide your patient care during clinical rotations. During clinicals, you can carry your concept map in your pocket or place it on your clipboard so you can refer to it often and update or revise it as necessary.

Teacher knows best

Concept mapping without tears

These guidelines can help you to learn how to quickly and easily create concept maps:
• Work quickly without pausing. Try to keep up with the flow of ideas. Don't stop to decide where something should go or to organize the material. Just get it down on paper. Ordering and analyzing are linear activities that can disrupt the mapping process.
• Write down everything you can think of without judging or editing—these activities can also disrupt the flow of concept mapping.
• If you come to a standstill, look over what you've done to see if you've left anything out.
• Confine the map to one page so it's easier to use.
• Print in capital letters for greater legibility. This also encourages you to keep the points brief.
• Initially, you may want to use color coding to group sections of the map. As you gain experience, you'll probably find that color coding isn't necessary.

On the case

Case study background

Mr. Jones is a 58-year-old male who was admitted to the medical-surgical floor with cholecystitis. The patient complains of pain in his epigastric area, nausea, and vomiting. His vital signs are as follows: heart rate 102 beats/minute, blood pressure 142/88 mm Hg, oral temperature 100.4° F, and respiratory rate 22 breaths/minute.

The patient rates his pain as an 8 on a scale of 0 to 10, with 10 being the most severe pain possible and 0 being the absence of pain. A nasogastric (NG) tube has been placed and is connected to low, intermittent wall suction, and an I.V. line with dextrose 5% in normal saline solution has been started at 75 ml/hour. Mr. Jones is scheduled for a laparoscopic cholecystectomy tomorrow.

Concept mapping exercise

Follow the steps outlined here to create a rough concept map for the care of Mr. Jones. Don't worry if you can't complete the entire care plan. This is just your first try. The answers can be found on page 21.

Steps

1. Assess the patient to collect clinical data.

2. Write the patient's name or initials, medical diagnosis, and chief complaint in the middle of a sheet of paper.

3. Write appropriate nursing diagnoses in boxes around the central box that contains the patient's name or initials and chief complaint. (*Hint:* One of the diagnoses should be *Acute pain.*)

4. Categorize assessment data under the appropriate nursing diagnoses.

5. Analyze the relationships among nursing diagnoses and draw lines to indicate these relationships.

6. On another piece of paper, identify patient goals, expected outcomes, and nursing interventions for the nursing diagnosis *Acute pain.* Or, instead of using another piece of paper, you can create additional boxes on your concept map for the goals, outcomes, and interventions and then link these boxes to the related nursing diagnoses.

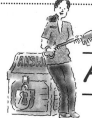

Answer key

Concept mapping exercise

Steps 1, 2, 3, 4, and 5

This concept map is one example of many possibilities for this patient. If you couldn't complete this concept map, don't worry. The remaining chapters in this book will walk you step-by-step through the process of creating a concept map that incorporates each stage of the nursing process.

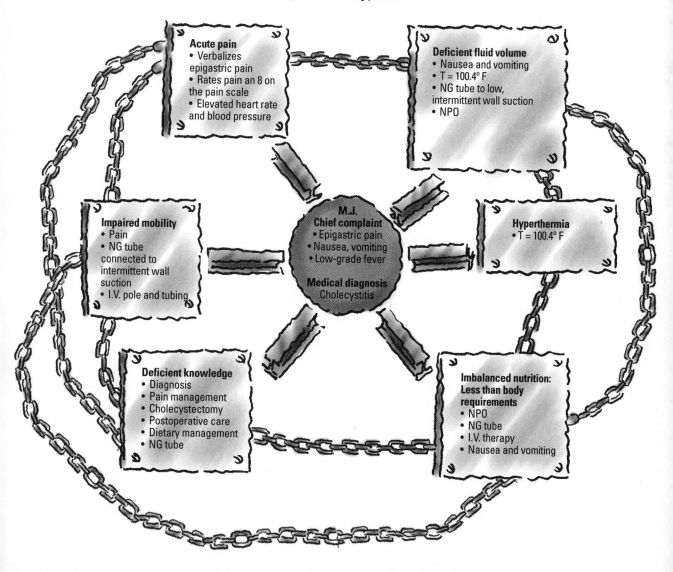

Acute pain
• Verbalizes epigastric pain
• Rates pain an 8 on the pain scale
• Elevated heart rate and blood pressure

Deficient fluid volume
• Nausea and vomiting
• T = 100.4° F
• NG tube to low, intermittent wall suction
• NPO

Impaired mobility
• Pain
• NG tube connected to intermittent wall suction
• I.V. pole and tubing

M.J.
Chief complaint
• Epigastric pain
• Nausea, vomiting
• Low-grade fever

Medical diagnosis
Cholecystitis

Hyperthermia
• T = 100.4° F

Deficient knowledge
• Diagnosis
• Pain management
• Cholecystectomy
• Postoperative care
• Dietary management
• NG tube

Imbalanced nutrition: Less than body requirements
• NPO
• NG tube
• I.V. therapy
• Nausea and vomiting

Step 6

Here's an example of a goal, expected outcomes, and nursing interventions for the nursing diagnosis *Acute pain*:

• *Nursing diagnosis:* Acute pain related to inflammation of the gallbladder as evidenced by the patient reporting pain rating as an 8 on a 0-to-10 scale

– *Nursing priority:* Pain control

• *Expected outcome:* Patient's self-reported pain level is reduced to 3 on a 0-to-10 scale within 2 hours of initiation of prescribed analgesics.

Nursing interventions	Evaluation
Assess pain using pain scale.	*This section will include the patient's responses to the interventions on the left.*
Medicate patient for pain, according to the practitioner's orders.	
Instruct patient on use of patient-controlled analgesia, if appropriate.	
Position patient for comfort.	
Use techniques of relaxation, meditation, or guided imagery.	

Assessment

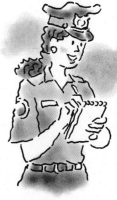

Just the facts

In this chapter, you'll learn:

♦ the components of a complete health assessment

♦ techniques and formats for gathering and organizing assessment data

♦ tips for reviewing a patient's chart for assessment data

♦ the steps for creating a concept map using assessment information.

A look at assessment

The first step in the nursing process, assessment involves data collection to identify the patient's actual and potential health problems and needs. The goal is to gather as much information about your patient as possible. Using these data, you'll identify his needs, formulate nursing diagnoses, establish expected outcomes, and identify interventions to help achieve those expected outcomes. You'll also set objective criteria to evaluate the effectiveness of your interventions.

> Think of the nursing assessment as a fact-finding mission.

Can I read that back to you?

Be sure to double-check, clarify, or restate the information you've collected to make sure that it's accurate and complete. Validating the data helps you avoid misinterpretation. Remember, if your assessment is incorrect or incomplete, the nursing diagnoses you formulate are likely to be incorrect as well or you may overlook a problem and neglect to formulate a diagnosis for it.

Also, to make sure that the data you've gathered accurately reflect the patient's life experiences and living patterns, maintain an objective, nonjudgmental approach during assessment.

Complete vs. focused assessment

Depending on the situation and time constraints, your assessment may be complete or focused.

You complete me

A *complete* assessment provides comprehensive baseline information. Typically, it's conducted when the patient is admitted. Student nurses are generally expected to perform a complete assessment as part of their learning experience.

Hocus focus

A *focused* assessment generally is problem- or need-oriented. During this assessment, focus on evaluating for specific problems or concerns that have already been identified and are being tracked by the health care team until they're resolved.

Typically, you'll perform a focused assessment after the patient has been admitted and undergone a complete assessment—for example, during initial shift assessment or change of assignment, whenever the patient has a new complaint or a change in condition, or when you're evaluating the results of an intervention.

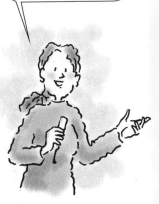

What did the care plan say to the assessment findings? You complete me!

Components of a complete health assessment

A complete health assessment includes the:
- nursing history
- physical assessment
- review of laboratory and diagnostic test results
- review of other available health information.

First impressions

Assessment begins as soon as you meet your patient. Perhaps without even being aware of it, you're already noting such aspects as his skin color, speech patterns, and body position. Your education as a nurse gives you the ability to organize and interpret these data. As you move on to conduct the formal nursing assessment, you'll collect data in a more structured way. The findings you collect from your assessment may be subjective or objective. (See *Subjective versus objective findings.*)

Group dynamics

When evaluating the assessment data, you'll start to recognize significant points and ask pertinent questions. You'll probably find

Teacher knows best

Subjective versus objective findings

Keep in mind that assessment findings fall into two broad categories: subjective and objective.

Subjective data

Subjective assessment data represents the perception or reality experienced by the person reporting the information. It may come directly from the patient or indirectly from family members, caregivers, or other health care providers. For example, when you ask a patient to rate his pain on a scale of 0 to 10, you're asking him to quantify his personal perception of the severity of his pain. Even indirect data can provide clues that could prove vital to your patient's care. In some cases—for instance, if your patient is physically or mentally incapable of answering questions or providing information—such third-party sources are crucial to your assessment.

Objective data

Objective data come from the physical examination through inspection, percussion, palpation, and auscultation. Use physical findings to verify the subjective findings you've gathered from the patient's health history. For example, diminished breath sounds heard on auscultation of the lower lobes of the lungs (objective data) support the patient's report of "having trouble breathing" (subjective data).

yourself starting to group related bits of significant assessment data into clusters that give you clues about your patient's problem and prompt additional questions. For instance, if the data suggest a pattern of poor nutrition, you should ask questions that will help elicit the cause, such as:

• Do you have a poor appetite?
• Do you eat most meals alone?
• Do you have enough money to buy food?

On the other hand, if the patient reports frequent nausea, you should suspect that this may be the cause of his poor nutrition. Therefore, you'd ask questions to elicit more information about this symptom, such as:

• Do you feel nauseated after meals? Before meals?
• Do any of your medications upset your stomach?

History

The nursing history requires you to collect information about the patient's:

• biographic data
• current physical and emotional complaints
• past medical history

- past and current ability to perform activities of daily living (ADLs)
- availability of support systems, effectiveness of past coping patterns, and perceived stressors
- socioeconomic factors affecting preventive health practices and compliance with medical recommendations
- spiritual and cultural practices, wishes, or concerns
- family patterns of illness.

Biographic data

Begin your history by obtaining biographic data from the patient. Do this before you begin gathering details about his health. Ask the patient his name, address, telephone number, birth date, age, marital status, religion, and nationality. Find out who the patient lives with and get the name and number of a person to contact in case of an emergency. Also ask the patient about his health care, including the name of his primary practitioner and his mode of transportation to practitioner visits. Finally, ask the patient if he has an advance directive and, if not, if he wants more information on advance directives.

   If the patient can't furnish accurate information, ask him for the name of a friend or relative who can. Always document the source of the information you collect as well as whether an interpreter was necessary.

Current complaints

To explore the patient's current complaints, ask the patient why he's seeking health care. Patient complaints provide valuable data immediately. When you explore these initial complaints, you may uncover crucial additional information.

Digging in the dirt

Record the patient's complaints in his own words. Ask him to describe the problem in detail, including any suspected cause. Keep in mind that, in many cases, presenting signs and symptoms are the tip of the iceberg. You must use your skills and knowledge to uncover facts about what's really going on. Obtaining a thorough patient history is one way to do this.

Past medical history

Ask the patient about past and current medical problems. Typical questions include:
- Have you ever been hospitalized? If so, when and why?
- Did you have any childhood illnesses?

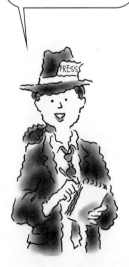

Recording your patient's complaints in his own words is good nursing practice. You can quote me on that!

• Are you currently being treated for any problem, such as hypertension or diabetes? If so, for what problem and who is your practitioner?
• Have you ever had surgery? If so, when and why?
• Are you allergic to anything in the environment or to any drugs or foods? If so, what kind of allergic reaction do you have?
• Are you taking medications, including over-the-counter (OTC) preparations, such as aspirin, vitamins, or cough syrup? If so, how much do you take and how often do you take it? Do you use home remedies such as homemade ointments? Do you use herbal preparations or take dietary supplements? Do you use other alternative or complementary therapies, such as acupuncture, massage, or chiropractic?
• Do you have any pain? If so, how would you rate your pain on a 0-to-10 pain scale? What aggravates or relieves your pain? How long have you had it?

Activities of daily living

Find out about your patient's ability to perform ADLs by asking him to describe his typical day. The types of information you seek should include:
• appetite, special diets, food allergies, and meal preparation
• urinary and bowel elimination habits
• exercise and sleep habits and any aids required for sleep
• work and leisure activities
• use of tobacco, alcohol, and other drugs.
   Also be sure to elicit the patient's view of how the present illness has affected his usual performance of ADLs.

Support systems and stressors

Because illness doesn't occur in isolation, you also need to ask about other aspects of your patient's life, including the availability of support systems and perceived stressors, when you collect your history data. These other life factors can enhance or complicate a patient's condition or affect his recovery.

Thank you for being a friend

For instance, lack of social support can affect a patient's physical well-being and influence patient outcomes. In addition to family members, a patient's social support system may include friends, coworkers, community agencies, avocational groups, and clergy who provide assistance in times of anxiety or crisis.
   You can begin your evaluation of your patient's support system by asking the patient, "Who's with you today?" or "How did you

get here today?" Other questions that elicit information about the patient's support system include:
- Is anyone available to assist you at home, if needed?
- Is the emotional support you receive from family and friends adequate?

More intimate details of the patient's social support system are usually best obtained in ongoing interactions during caregiving activities or as you and the patient begin to discuss discharge plans. As appropriate, weave the information you obtain about your patient's support system into the care plan.

Stress marks

Emotional, social, and physical demands on the body cause stress. The amount of stress a patient experiences can affect his physiologic and psychological health. To elicit information about your patient's stress level and methods of coping with stress, ask:
- what situations he finds stressful
- how he responds physically to stress
- what he does when he feels stress
- whether stress affects his family relationships
- if he thinks stress affects his health.

Also, inquire about potential stressors, such as recent losses or setbacks, spiritual concerns, difficulties with self-care or normal ADLs, and exposure to abuse (see *Asking about abuse*). These may be important clues that help you formulate a care plan.

Asking about abuse

A history of abuse is an important aspect of a patient's psychosocial history. Remember that anyone can be a victim of abuse, including a boyfriend or girlfriend, a spouse, an elderly person, a child, or a parent. In addition, abuse can occur in many forms, including physical, psychological, emotional, and sexual abuse.

When taking a health history, you should ask two questions to explore abuse:
- When do you feel safe at home?
- When do you not feel safe at home?

Reaction time
Even when you don't immediately suspect an abusive situation, be aware of how your patient reacts to open-ended questions. Is the patient defensive, hostile, confused, or frightened? Assess how the patient interacts with you and others. Does he seem withdrawn or frightened or show other inappropriate behavior? Keep his reactions in mind when you perform your physical assessment.

Remember to report
Remember, if the patient tells you about any type of abuse, you're obligated to report it. Inform the patient that you must report the incident to local authorities.

Socioeconomic factors

The patient's socioeconomic status can directly affect health behaviors by determining the financial resources available for health
care and a healthful lifestyle, including adequate housing, clothing, and nutrition. For example, a patient whose insurance plan
doesn't reimburse routine health screening and physical examina-
tions usually seeks health care only for illness. Similarly, a patient
whose financial resources barely meet basic needs is less likely to
use services or products designed to promote or maintain health.

Insurance plan

To assess health-related socioeconomic factors, find out if your
patient has health insurance and, if so, whether insurance pays for
a routine physical examination or other screening procedures.
Also find out whether the patient is receiving financial aid and
whether his income is sufficient to pay for housing, food, and
clothing.

Spiritual and cultural influences

Some patients attach great importance to their spiritual and religious beliefs. Spirituality (one's personal definition of the purpose
and meaning of life and the world) may assign meaning to individual and community life, guide daily behavior and lifestyle, define
acceptable health care, and influence attitudes toward illness and
death.

Divine thing

Religion is the component of spirituality that includes particular
practices related to a belief in a divine power. A religious system
usually embraces more specific beliefs, including prescribed behaviors, rituals, or practices. A patient's health beliefs and practices may be linked closely to religion.

Culture club

A patient's cultural background can also profoundly influence his
views of life and death, health beliefs, health and dietary habits,
roles, relationships, and family dynamics. For example, patients
from some cultures avoid seeking health care or taking responsibility for changing unhealthful behaviors because they feel power-
less to control their illness, which they may consider punishment
for some wrongdoing. To find out about your patient's spiritual
and cultural influences, ask these questions:
• Do you have religious or cultural beliefs that affect your diet or
health practices?
• Would you like me to contact any religious affiliation for you?

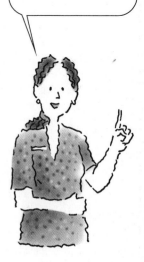

When assessing
your patient's
spiritual beliefs, don't
let your own beliefs
color your attitude.
Remember to remain
nonjudgmental.

Assessing cultural influences can bring health-related factors to light and identify culturally related strengths, such as a strong support system.

Lost in translation?

If the patient has a language barrier, talk with your manager or the family to assist you in finding an interpreter. When you first interact with the patient with an interpreter present, explain the facility's basic routines and establish a functional method of communicating about important health issues, such as pain, constipation, nausea, or other common symptoms. This is also a good time to verify that the patient understands use of the call bell and any treatments or restrictions ordered.

Show a little respect

Being observant, open, and interested is commonly the best way to learn about other people's spiritual and cultural viewpoints. Whether you're asking questions or responding to patient queries, be careful to avoid making assumptions about people who might be ethnically or culturally different from you. A simple question opener such as, "Would you be comfortable if I…?" can demonstrate your respect for the patient's feelings and your willingness to adapt your care to the patient's needs.

Family history

Questioning the patient about his family's health is a good way to uncover his risk of having certain illnesses. (See *All in the family history.*)

All in the family history

Being aware of patterns of illness in families can help you understand genetic risk factors, determine the influence of these events on the attitudes of your patient, and plan effective interventions. For example, a 49-year-old male with a family history of several male deaths from heart attack before age 50 who experiences chest pain may be significantly more afraid or hopeless than a peer with a similar complaint but no early male cardiac deaths in his family.

In some clinical settings, you may not have access to a family medical history because it's obtained by the practitioner but isn't immediately available to you. In this case, obtain a brief history of relevant illness in the patient's parents, siblings and, when indicated, grandparents. Typical questions include:
• Are your mother, father, and siblings living?
• If not, how old were they when they died? What were the causes of their deaths?
• If they're alive, do they have diabetes, high blood pressure, heart disease, asthma, cancer, sickle cell anemia, hemophilia, cataracts, glaucoma, or other illnesses?

Physical examination

During the physical examination, you obtain data using your five senses—sight, hearing, touch, smell, and feel. A complete examination includes a general survey, measurement of vital signs, height and weight measurements, and assessment of all organs and body systems. (See *Examining the goals of a physical examination.*) This type of examination is appropriate for periodic health checks. Of course, in many cases, you won't have time for a complete examination and will need to focus on particular complaints or health problems.

General survey

The general survey provides vital information about the patient's behavior and health status. During your first contact with the patient, expect to receive a steady stream of impressions—most of which are visual. The patient's sex, race, and approximate age will generally be obvious. Because some health concerns may relate to these factors, be sure to note them.

Also note less-obvious factors that can contribute to an overall impression, including:
- signs of distress
- facial characteristics
- body type, posture, and movements
- speech
- dress
- grooming and personal hygiene
- style of interacting with others.

Teacher knows best

Examining the goals of a physical examination

During the physical examination, keep in mind that your goal as a nurse is to identify signs, symptoms, and problems for which the patient needs nursing interventions. In other words, the data you collect should lead you to formulate a nursing diagnosis—not a medical diagnosis. The nurse's focus is always on patient processes.

Medical practitioners (such as doctors, nurse practitioners, and physician assistants), on the other hand, use a method called *differential diagnosis* to arrive at a medical diagnosis. After identifying signs and symptoms, they systematically eliminate related diagnoses until they identify and substantiate a precise diagnosis by objective means, such as radiologic or laboratory findings. The practitioner's focus is the disease processes.

Meaningful collaboration among practitioners and nurses leads to health care that maximizes the patient's health and quality of life or preserves his comfort and dignity in death.

Summarize

When you've completed the survey, document your initial impressions of the patient in a one-paragraph statement—a summary that gives an overall picture to guide your subsequent examination.

Physical examination techniques

To perform the physical examination, you'll use four basic techniques—inspection, palpation, percussion, and auscultation.

All eyes on inspection

Inspection, or critical observation, is the most frequently used assessment technique. Performed correctly, it also reveals more than the other techniques. But incomplete or hasty inspection may neglect important details or yield false or misleading findings.

To ensure accurate, useful information, approach inspection in a careful, unhurried manner. Pay close attention to details as you assess each body system, observing for color, size, location, movement, texture, symmetry, odors, and sounds. Try to draw logical conclusions from the findings.

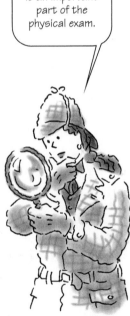

Don't forget that inspection is an important part of the physical exam.

Palpation points

During palpation, you touch the patient's body with your hands, using various degrees of pressure to feel pulsations and vibrations, locate body structures, and assess such characteristics as size, texture, warmth, mobility, and tenderness. Palpation allows you to detect a pulse, muscle rigidity, enlarged lymph nodes, skin dryness, organ tenderness, or breast lumps as well as measure chest expansion and contraction during respiration.

Percussion discussion

During percussion, you tap your fingers or hands quickly and sharply against body surfaces (usually the chest and abdomen) to produce sounds, detect tenderness, or assess reflexes. Percussion for sound (the most common goal) helps locate organ borders, identify organ shape and position, and determine if an organ is solid or filled with fluid or gas.

Listen closely

Auscultation involves listening to body sounds—especially those produced by the heart, lungs, blood vessels, stomach, and intestines. For all but the most pronounced body sounds, you'll need a stethoscope to auscultate.

Diagnostic testing data

Make sure that you know how to access the patient's laboratory and other diagnostic test results. In most record-keeping systems, laboratory results are printed or electronically formatted on forms that specify what laboratory performed the test, the normal range of values for that test, the patient's test value, and where that value lies in relation to the normal range. Remember that "normal" values for many tests vary somewhat between different laboratories, depending on the specific equipment or testing techniques they use. In a student nursing care plan, always cite the range listed for the laboratory performing the test.

Other test results may be filed by type or located by date of service. Radiology, nuclear scanning, computed tomography, magnetic resonance imaging, and ultrasound results commonly are kept together. Endoscopic and biopsy reports may be filed separately, with the report containing a section on the procedure process as well as the specific findings. Electrocardiograms are commonly kept together for ease of comparison.

Supporting role

Nurses not only need to be aware of what tests the patient has had and the results, but should have an understanding of the disease process and what these results may mean. Patients may be understandably anxious about the details of preparing for or going through a particular test, how soon results will be available, and what these results mean. The nurse is responsible for teaching and preparing the patient and then identifying and responding to post-test complications or reactions. The practitioner is responsible for conveying test results and implications to the patient, but nurses are commonly asked to review and clarify the information provided as the patient thinks through what he has been told.

Other health information in the patient's chart

The patient's chart is an excellent source of assessment data. Always review it carefully, including assessments made by other health care team members, such as emergency department (ED) staff, the admitting practitioner, consulting medical specialists, other nursing staff and advanced practice consultants, dietitians, physical or other specialty therapy personnel, pharmacy consultants, social service workers, and discharge planners. The practitioner's history and physical examination findings can guide your questioning during assessment. If appropriate, you should attempt to corroborate these findings during the nursing assessment. If your assessment findings differ, report your findings as appropriate.

Medication use

Be sure to review your patient's current medication use. Ask about prescription drugs, OTC drugs, and herbal remedies. List these medications on the patient's chart when he's admitted to the facility. Medications that are prescribed during hospitalization are listed on a medication administration record (MAR). Look closely at the details of each drug order.

Get to know your patient's medication list inside and out. It may affect your care plan. Getting to know you...

Look before you leap

Before your clinical rotation or first patient contact, check your patient's list of prescribed drugs and their dosages and make sure that you know what adverse reactions and interactions these drugs could cause. Also find out if the patient understands the purpose of each drug; this will help determine if he needs additional teaching during hospitalization or at discharge. If appropriate, ask about the patient's previous medication use as well, find out if he experienced adverse reactions, and ask about recreational drug use.

If you question a drug, dosage, or route listed on the MAR, double-check the original order in the medical record first, and then call the pharmacy or practitioner as appropriate. In the home care setting, check the labels on the patient's prescriptions and call the pharmacy or the practitioner to validate discrepancies between the labels, the patient's statements, and the physician orders in the nursing record.

Overdose of drug data

For educational purposes, nursing instructors commonly have students complete a data sheet on all drugs assigned to the patient. (See *Everything you always wanted to know about drugs but were afraid of forgetting* and *Resources for reliable drug information*, pages 37 and 38.)

Medical procedure data

Review the medical procedures scheduled for your patient. Knowing which procedures the patient is scheduled for can help you anticipate potential problems and alert you to postprocedure signs and symptoms to watch for.

For example...

If the patient is scheduled for myelography, you would expect to verify the allergy history, looking particularly for an allergy to iodine or other contrast materials, and notify the referring practitioner and radiologist of new information. You would also expect to explain to the patient what's going to happen before, during, and after the procedure, including transfer to the radiology suite,

(Text continues on page 38.)

Everything you always wanted to know about drugs but were afraid of forgetting

To help you learn and retain important information about the multitude of drugs you'll be administering, student nursing care plans commonly contain a detailed section on the drugs the assigned patient is taking. Here are typical types of information you might collect on each drug and a sample entry.

Information required	Example
Generic name (trade name)	• Lisinopril (Prinivil, Zestril)
Class (pharmacologic, therapeutic, or both)	• *Pharmacologic:* Angiotensin-converting enzyme (ACE) inhibitor • *Therapeutic:* Antihypertensive
Action	• Lowers blood pressure by suppressing the renin-angiotensin-aldosterone system • Blocks the enzyme that converts angiotensin I to angiotensin II, which also decreases aldosterone production • Causes decreased blood pressure from less vasoconstriction, a small increase in potassium, and some sodium and fluid loss
Dose (normal and patient's)	• *Normal:* Initially, 5 mg daily when patient is also on a thiazide diuretic; usual effective dosage 20 to 40 mg daily; maximum dosage 80 mg daily • *Patient:* 10 mg daily (also on hydrochlorothiazide)
Specific therapeutic use (this patient)	• Lower blood pressure below 120/80 mm Hg because diuretic alone was insufficient
Contraindications and precautions	• Contraindicated in patients hypersensitive to or with a history of angioedema from ACE inhibitors • Contraindicated in women who are in their last two trimesters of pregnancy • Use cautiously in patients with impaired renal function (may need to adjust dose) • Use cautiously in patients at risk for hyperkalemia, heart failure (use only when other drugs are ineffective), or salt or volume depletion • Use cautiously in women who are breast-feeding • Rare but life-threatening adverse reactions: hyperkalemia, angioedema, anaphylaxis, pancytopenia
Major adverse effects	• Common adverse reactions: dizziness, fatigue, headache, insomnia: orthostatic hypotension; nasal congestion; diarrhea, nausea; muscle cramps; dry, persistent, tickling, nonproductive cough (most common reason for stopping drug due to side effects)

(continued)

Everything you always wanted to know about drugs but were afraid of forgetting (continued)

Information required	Example
Drug or food interactions	• Capsaicin (Capsin, Zostrix): may worsen cough • Digoxin (Lanoxin): may increase digoxin levels, risking toxicity • Diuretics: may cause excessively low blood pressure • Indomethacin (Indocin): may interfere with blood pressure lowering effect of lisinopril • Potassium-sparing diuretics, potassium supplements: may increase risk of hyper-kalemia • Thiazide diuretics: may decrease potassium loss caused by these diuretics • Insulins, oral antidiabetics: may increase risk of hypoglycemia • Lithium carbonate (Lithobid): may increase lithium levels, risking toxicity • Phenothiazines: may increase blood-pressure-lowering effects, risking hypotension • Licorice: may cause sodium retention and increased blood pressure counteracting the effects of lisinopril
Effects on laboratory test results	• May increase potassium, blood urea nitrogen, serum creatinine, and liver function test levels, including bilirubin
Nursing implications (including route of administration)	• Assess white blood cell count with differential, serum potassium level, and kidney and liver function before starting the drug and periodically thereafter. • Monitor for adverse effects and drug interactions. • Give orally without regard to meals (although use with meals may decrease GI adverse effects). • Determine if the patient is pregnant or may become pregnant. Notify the practitioner as needed and tell the patient of the risks.
Patient teaching	• Teach the patient to immediately call or see a practitioner if swelling of eyes, face, lips, or tongue with difficulty breathing appears (most common with first dose of drug). • Instruct the patient that light-headedness may occur, especially during the first few days of treatment; to rise slowly to avoid this effect; to notify the practitioner; and to stop the drug and call the practitioner promptly if fainting occurs. • Tell the patient to watch for signs of infection, such as fever, sore throat, productive cough, and poorly healing wounds and to notify the practitioner if any of these signs occur. • Teach women of child-bearing age to use effective contraception and to stop the drug if pregnancy occurs. • Inform the patient of the importance of regular blood pressure monitoring and laboratory testing by the practitioner. Also, teach about the use of a home blood pressure monitoring device, if appropriate.

Resources for reliable drug information

In some cases, you might find it difficult to locate all the information you need to know about a drug or an herbal product. For example, you might not be able to find information on the off-label uses of drugs and on over-the-counter (OTC) drugs and herbs in your standard drug reference.

Off-label uses

The U.S. Food and Drug Administration (FDA) is responsible for issuing permits for the sale of all prescription and nonprescription drugs in the United States as well as approving the content of each drug's product label (package insert). However, practitioners aren't restricted to prescribing drugs only according to their approved product labels. Research is constantly being done on "off-label" uses. For example, certain anticonvulsants, such as oxcarbazepine (Trileptal), are commonly prescribed for patients with bipolar disorder who can't tolerate or don't respond to lithium carbonate (Lithobid), even though the FDA hasn't yet approved these drugs for this indication. Observation by prescribers in clinical practice revealed that patients taking the drug for partial seizures also experienced control of their bipolar symptoms. Scholarly articles spread the word, leading more prescribers to try the drug with their patients. Now research is in progress to meet the standards for FDA approval of this drug for this use. However, you might not find this information in your everyday drug reference.

Over-the-counter drugs, herbs, and supplements

Information on OTC drugs, herbs, and supplements (including vitamins and minerals) also might not appear in your usual drug reference. However, you'll need good resource material about these products. The fact that they're readily available leads some of these products to be dangerously used and abused. Some patients assume that if a drug is sold without a prescription, it's completely safe to use, even overuse, regardless of the warnings on the label. A good resource can help you determine all the risks of improper use, expand your understanding of potential adverse effects, alert you to potential interactions with other drugs and herbs, and help you plan patient teaching.

Because the FDA doesn't currently regulate herbal products, these products can vary widely in the doses they deliver. Nurses, pharmacists, and prescribers need to keep up-to-date with the latest research on herbal preparations, including what medical conditions can be helped by various herbs, what dosages appear to be beneficial, what dosages appear to be

toxic, and what adverse effects or drug interactions might occur. Being attuned to good sources of reliable information can assist you in caring for your patients.

Finding reliable references

When researching drug information, remember to check the date of publication. Many nursing and practitioner references are updated yearly, but not all. Drug product labels are only updated when new indications or dosage forms are approved or new warnings are required by the FDA.

The resources listed here are available to provide you with reliable drug and herb information.

Prescription drugs

• The drug product label is the most valid source of FDA-approved information. However, the label doesn't list off-label drug uses.
• Product labels are available at the FDA's web site (*www.accessdata.fda.gov*) and drug manufacturers' web sites (search by trade name or company).
• Companies that manufacture older generic drugs may no longer make the drug product label readily available. Reputable online pharmacy web sites, such as *www.drugs.com* and *www.rxlist.com,* are good sources of information about these products.
• Several pharmacist- and practitioner-oriented drug reference books, such as *Facts and Comparisons,* can generally be found in your school library. These resources usually provide more-accessible formats and a wider range of information—such as off-label uses—than product labels.
• Many nurses prefer to use a nursing drug reference book for day-to-day information geared to their needs. Such books as the *Nursing Drug Handbook* (and companion web site *www.NDHnow.com*) or *Springhouse Nurse's Drug Guide* (geared toward students) can be invaluable for checking nursing considerations and patient teaching information in addition to providing essential information on indications, dosages, con-

(continued)

Resources for reliable drug information (continued)

traindications and cautions, therapeutic and pharmacologic effects, and adverse reactions.

• Specialty references, such as *Dangerous Drug Interactions* by Lippincott Williams & Wilkins and *Patient Drug Facts* by Facts & Comparisons, can also be useful in developing teaching plans.

Over-the-counter drugs

• Some information on OTC (nonprescription) drugs is available from prescription drug sources because these drugs are commonly sold in higher-dose, prescription products.

• Specialty nonprescription drug references, such as *Nonprescription Drug Therapy* by Facts & Comparisons, are also available.

• The U.S. National Library of Medicine's and the National Institutes of Health's (NIH) MedlinePlus (*www.medlineplus.gov*) and the online RxList (*www.rxlist.com*) also provide some information about these drugs.

Herbal products

• The NIH and U.S. Library of Medicine also sponsor a web site (*www.nlm.nih.gov/medlineplus/druginformation.html*) containing independent information on herbal products, including the latest research findings.

• *The Review of Natural Products* by Facts & Comparisons, which may be available in your school library, is an example of a reliable publication from providers of prescription information.

• The nursing-based resource *Nursing Herbal Medicine Handbook* provides nursing considerations and patient-teaching information in addition to the standard information.

---

and instruct him about procedure restrictions, including the need to:

• withhold solid foods and certain medications before the test
• void right before the test
• remove any jewelry
• maintain a side-lying, fetal-type position during injection of the contrast medium into the spinal canal by the radiologist just before the test.

Similarly, if the patient has just undergone a procedure involving anesthetics or other medications, you would know to assess for adverse reactions to these agents.

Admitting medical diagnosis

You should also review the patient's medical diagnosis. Determine if your patient's current complaints and assessment findings match his admitting diagnosis. If you uncover new information, report it to the practitioner because these new findings may affect the treatment plan. Make sure you understand the meaning and implications of your patient's medical diagnosis—including its pathophysiology, signs and symptoms, required diagnostic tests, treatments, complications, preparation for procedures, and post-procedure care. This information helps you focus your assessment.

Special consideration

If your patient is diagnosed with ulcerative colitis, for instance, you would realize that he's more prone to develop anemia due to internal bleeding. Consequently, you would be sure to monitor his hematology reports, check his vital signs frequently, and observe elimination patterns and changes. On the other hand, for a patient admitted with diabetes mellitus, you would stay alert for signs and symptoms of hypoglycemia or hyperglycemia.

Data collection and organization

Every nurse must know how to collect and organize patient data in a meaningful format. Doing this helps you formulate correct nursing diagnoses and allows other health care team members to readily understand the data you've documented.

In your educational process, you are often asked to organize your information by functional health patterns. In the clinical setting, many different types of integrated or specialty assessment database formats may be used, according to the regulations and specific requirements for that facility.

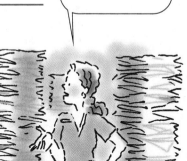

The data you collect on your patient can be overwhelming. Good thing that there are systems for organizing all these data.

Gordon's functional health patterns

To organize and analyze the patient data you collect, you may want to use the functional health patterns and rating scale proposed in 1987 by Marjory Gordon. Gordon's functional health categories include:
- health perception and management
- nutrition and metabolism
- elimination
- activity and exercise
- cognition and perception
- sleep and rest
- self-perception and self-concept
- sexuality and reproduction
- roles and relationships
- coping and stress management
- values and beliefs.

These 11 categories provide a framework for a systematic, standardized approach to data collection.

You can use Gordon's functional health patterns to obtain a nursing history from the patient's perspective through a series of specific questions. These patterns are flexible and adaptable and can be used for patients in various states of health, from different age-groups, and in different clinical settings. Gordon's functional health patterns have also become an integral part of many nursing database documentation systems.

Deciphering code

To document your patient's functional health patterns, you'll assign a code based on a five-point scale that rates the ability of the patient to function independently. (See *Assigning functional level codes.*) By focusing on each health pattern in turn, you can better evaluate your patient's overall level of health and well-being.

Health perception and management

To obtain data about the health perception and management pattern, ask questions that help determine the patient's:
• perception of his level of health
• detrimental habits, such as smoking or excessive alcohol use
• actual or potential problems related to safety and health management or the need for home modifications or continued care at home.

Activity and exercise

When evaluating the patient's activity and exercise pattern, assess:
• the patient's ability to manage normal ADLs that require energy expenditure, including self-care, exercise, and leisure time
• major body systems involved with activity and exercise (respiratory, cardiovascular, and musculoskeletal systems).

Nutrition and metabolism

To assess nutrition and metabolism, ask the patient questions about:
• food and fluid consumption relative to metabolic needs
• adequacy of nourishment
• dietary habits and preferences
• problems related to fluid balance, tissue integrity, adequate nutrition, and immunologic defenses
• GI problems.

Elimination

To assess your patient's elimination pattern, ask questions related to his excretory patterns (bowel, bladder, and skin) and check for such problems as incontinence, constipation, diarrhea, and urinary retention.

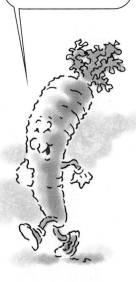

Gordon says that nutrition and metabolism are one of the 11 functional health categories.

Assigning functional level codes

Some facilities require nurses to assign codes during patient assessment to describe the patient's functional level according to Gordon's functional health patterns (as shown at right). This type of scale has been adapted to many settings and uses, particularly in long-term care assessments of activities of daily living. As a student, your instructor may also require you to grade the patient's functional level.

Grading system

If you're asked to assign functional level codes, you'll grade the functional level of the patient on a scale of 0 to 4 in each of the 11 categories described in the text. You'll also assign a code that most closely describes the patient's overall functional level.

Code name "Outcomes"

Functional levels can also be incorporated into your expected outcomes. To do this, you would include a reference to the functional level you expect the patient to attain as a result of your nursing interventions and other collaborative care. Say, for example, a patient is receiving rehabilitation after a hip fracture repair. Based on your initial assessment, you rate his functional mobility level as 3 because he requires supervision to stand up and walk safely with a walker. Your expected outcome statement might read: "Attains functional mobility level of 1 as demonstrated by standing up and walking 15' with a cane, unassisted, by discharge." You'll read more about writing outcome statements in chapter 4, Planning.

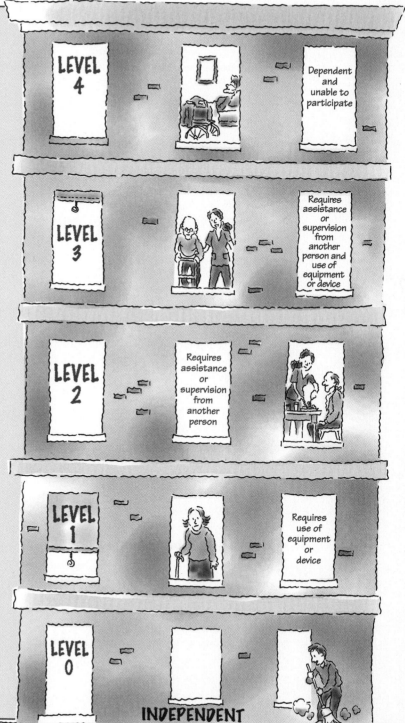

Sleep and rest

When assessing the patient's sleep and rest pattern, inquire about:
• sleep, rest, and relaxation practices
• dysfunctional sleep patterns, fatigue, and responses to sleep deprivation.

Cognition and perception

To assess cognition and perception, evaluate the patient's:
• ability to comprehend and use information
• sensory and neurologic functions
• sensory experiences, such as pain and altered sensory input.

Self-perception and self-concept

To assess your patient's self-perception and self-concept, evaluate:
• attitudes toward self, including identity, body image, self-worth, and self-esteem
• response to threats to self-concept.

Sexuality and reproduction

To assess the patient's sexuality and reproduction pattern, evaluate:
• satisfaction or dissatisfaction with sexuality patterns and reproductive functions
• sexuality concerns.

Roles and relationships

To assess your patient's roles and relationships, evaluate:
• roles in the world and relationships with others
• satisfaction with roles
• role strain
• dysfunctional relationships.

Coping and stress management

Explore your patient's coping and stress management pattern by asking questions about his:
• perception of stress and coping strategies
• support systems
• symptoms of stress
• effectiveness of coping strategies in terms of stress tolerance.

Values and beliefs

To assess the patient's values and beliefs, evaluate:
• religious or spiritual orientation
• goals and values that guide decisions.

Integrated and specialty database formats

For consistency, most health care facilities require that staff document assessment findings using standardized formats. Typically, history and physical findings are on the same form. The purpose of using a standardized format is to provide a comprehensive, consistent, understandable framework for nursing data. (See *Joint Commission standards for initial assessments.*) Standardized formats enhance information exchange and communication among staff members and, when necessary, among health care facilities. However, when a standardized format is used, nurses typically adapt their assessment techniques to the flow of the form. (See *Integrated admission database form*, pages 44 to 47.)

Custom or generic?

Some facilities use assessment forms customized for their particular needs; others use more generic forms developed by outside vendors. Some standardized forms are designed to promote closer monitoring and evaluation of patient status trends, patterns, and longitudinal observations and changes. They're especially useful in critical care areas, where the patient's status can change in mere moments.

Digital age

Health care providers are increasingly using computerized charting, handheld computers, and personal digital assistants to collect and organize real-time (or near real-time) patient information

(Text continues on page 48.)

Memory jogger

To remember Gordon's functional patterns, think of the slogan "Hey Nurse! Every Action Can Start, Stimulate, Stop, or Reverse your Care Victory!"

Health perception and management

Nutrition and metabolism

Elimination

Activity and exercise

Cognition and perception

Sleep and rest

Self-perception and self-concept

Sexuality and reproduction

Roles and relationships

Coping and stress management

Values and beliefs

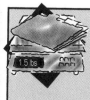

1.5 lbs

Weighing the evidence

Joint Commission standards for initial assessments

The Joint Commission has developed standards for the initial nursing assessment of patients. The commission determines its standards by examining the criteria of nursing professional organizations and relevant research. The Joint Commission standards state that the following items should be considered in an initial assessment:

• physical factors
• psychological, social, and cultural factors
• environmental factors
• self-care capabilities
• learning needs
• discharge planning needs
• input from the patient's family and friends, when appropriate.

Integrated admission database form

Most health care facilities use a multidisciplinary admission form. The sample form below has spaces that can be filled in by the nurse, physician, and other health care providers.

Name _Beatrice Perry_

Address _2 Clayton Street_

Dallas, Texas 55532

Admission Date _2 / 26 / 01_ Time _1345_

Admitted per: ____ Ambulatory

✔ Stretcher ____ Wheelchair

T _91_ P _92_ R _24_ BP _98 / 52_

Ht. _5'2"_ Wt. _225 lb_

(estimated/actual)

SECTION COMPLETED BY: _P. Lippman, CST_   **TIME:** _1350_

ORIENTATION TO ROOM/UNIT
POLICIES EXPLAINED
- ✔ Call light
- ✔ Bed oper.
- ✔ Phone
- ✔ Television
- ✔ Meals
- ___ Advance directive explained
- ___ Living will

- ___ Living will on chart
- ___ Valuables form completed
- ✔ Elec.
- ✔ Smoking
- ___ Side rails
- ✔ ID bracelet on
- ___ Visiting hours

Name and phone numbers of two people to call if necessary:

NAME	RELATIONSHIP	PHONE #
Mary Ryan	_daughter_	_234-555-2190_
Thomas Perry	_son_	_234-555-4785_

REASON FOR HOSPITALIZATION ____ (patient quote:) _I go numb in my (R) arm and leg_

ANTICIPATED DATE OF DISCHARGE: _2/28/01_

PREVIOUS HOSPITALIZATIONS: SURGERY/ILLNESS   DATE _1/15/01_

TIA

HEALTH PROBLEM	Yes	No	?
Arthritis		✔	
Blood problem (anemia, sickle cell, clotting, bleeding)		✔	
Cancer		✔	
Diabetes	✔		
Eye problems (cataracts, glaucoma)		✔	
Heart problem		✔	
Liver problem		✔	
Hiatal hernia		✔	
High blood pressure	✔		
HIV/AIDS		✔	
Kidney problem		✔	
Comments:			

HEALTH PROBLEM	Yes	No	?
Lung problem (Emphysema) Asthma, Bronchitis, TB, Pneumonia, Shortness of breath)	✔		
Stroke		✔	
Ulcers		✔	
Thyroid problem		✔	
Psychological disorder		✔	
Alcohol abuse		✔	
Drug abuse			
Drug(s)_____		✔	
Smoking	✔		
Other _____			

ALLERGIES: ☐ TAPE ☐ IODINE ☐ LATEX ☐ no known allergies

☐ FOOD:_____   ✔ DRUG: _Penicillin - Rash_

☐ BLOOD REACTION:_____   ☐ OTHER:_____

MEDICATIONS: _____

HERBAL PREPARATIONS: _____

INFORMATION RECEIVED FROM: **SECTION COMPLETED BY:**

✔ Patient ☐ Relative_____ ☐ Friend_____ ☐ Other_____   _Jill O'Brien, RN_   Date _2/26/01_ Time _1405_

Integrated admission database form *(continued)*

All assessment sections are to be completed by a professional nurse. Date __2/28/01__

Patient name: _Beatrice Perry_
Record number: ___554641___

GENERAL PHYSICAL APPEARANCE

✔ Clean _____ Disheveled

SKIN INTEGRITY: Indicate the location of any of the following on the chart to the right using the designated letter: a = rashes, b = lesions, c = significant bruises/ abrasions, d = burns, e = pressure sores, f = recent scars, g = presence of tubes/ appliances, h = other

Comments: _____b: ischemic leg ulcer (2 cm - healing)_____

PRESSURE SORE POTENTIAL ASSESSMENT

PARAMETERS	0	1	2	3	Score
Mental status	(Alert)	Lethargic	Semicomatose (Count as double)	Comatose (Count as double)	0
Activity	Ambulatory	(Needs help)	Chairfast	Bedfast	1
Mobility	Full	(Limited)	Very limited	Immobile	1
Incontinence	(None)	Occasional	Usually of urine	Total of urine and feces	0
Oral nutrition intake	Good	(Fair)	Poor	None	1
Oral fluid intake	(Good)	Fair	Poor	None	0
Predisposing diseases (diabetes, neuropathies, vascular disease, anemias)	Absent	Slight	Moderate	(Severe)	3
Patients with scores of 10 or above should be considered at risk.				Total	6

FALL-RISK ASSESSMENT

Impaired:
____ sensory function
____ urinary/GI function
____ mobility function
____ mental status

____ general debility/weakness
✔ history of recent falls/dizziness/blackouts
(automatically designates patient as prone-to-fall)
✔ prone-to-fall risk (indicated on nursing Kardex ___✔___)

NEUROLOGICAL

____ Dizziness   ____ Syncope   ____ Headache   ____ Blurred vision
____ Recent seizure   ✔ Numbness/tingling location: (R) arm and leg
LOC: ✔ Alert   ____ Lethargic   ____ Semicomatose   ____ Comatose
Mental Status: ✔ Oriented   ____ Confused   ____ Disoriented
Speech: ✔ Clear   ____ Slurred   ____ Garbled   ____ Aphasic

Neurological Checklist

	Right Arm	Left Arm	Right Leg	Left Leg	Right Pupil	Left Pupil	Pupil Reaction	Eyes Open	Best Verbal Response	Best Motor Response	Total
Coma Scale	+2/+4		+2/+4		5/6		↑	4	5	6	15

	Response	1	2	3	4	5	6
COMA SCALE CODE	EYES OPEN	Never	To Pain	To Sound	Sponta-neously		
	VERBAL	None	Incompre-hensible Sounds	Inappro-priate Words	Confused Conversa-tion	Oriented	
	MOTOR	None	Extension	Flexion Abnormal	Flexion Withdrawal	Localizes Pain	

+1: cannot move
+2: cannot move against gravity
+3: move against gravity
+4: move strongly against gravity

CODE
Pupils: mm
Extremities movement/strength
Pupil Reaction
- Reactive
- Nonreactive
D Dilated
C Constricted
> Greater than
< Less than
= Equal
= Sluggish

1 2 3 4 5 6 7

Comments: _numbness transient_

T. Jones, MD

BEHAVIORAL

Behavior: ✔ Cooperative   ____ Uncooperative   ____ Depressed
____ Restless   ____ Other
____ Combative   ✔ Anxious   ____ Unresponsive

Comments: _____
Religious/Spiritual beliefs: _Lutheran_
Pt. request to contact minister/priest/rabbi? ✔ Y ___ N
Name _Rev. William Lacy_ Phone # _234-555-8039_

PAIN

Pt. having pain at present? ___Y ✔N
Pt. had pain in last several months? ___Y ✔N
Rate pain on a scale of 0-10 (0 = no pain, 10 = severe pain) _____
Pain location _____ Quality _____

Radiation ___Y ___N Duration _____
What aggravates pain? _____ What alleviates pain? _____
Effects on ADLs _____
Pt. pain goals _____

(continued)

Integrated admission database form *(continued)*

Patient name: _Beatrice Perry_
Record number: _554697_   Date _2/28/01_

CARDIOVASCULAR

Skin Color: ___Normal ___Flushed ___Pale ✔Cyanotic
Apical Pulse: ___Regular ✔Irregular ___Pacemaker: Type _____ Rate _____ _bilat. weak lower extremities_
Peripheral Pulses: ✔ Present ___Equal ✔ Weak ___Absent Comments: _____
Specify: R____radial ___ pedal L ___radial ___pedal
Comments:____
Edema: ___No ✔Yes _+/ bilat. pretibial_ Numbness: ___No ✔Yes Site: _Ⓡ arm and leg_
Chest Pain: ✔No ___Yes___ P_____ Q_____ R_____ S_____ T_____
Family Cardiac History: ___No ✔Yes Telemetry Monitor: ___No ✔Yes rhythm _normal sinus_
Comments:____

PULMONARY

Respirations: ✔ Regular ___Irregular ___Shortness of breath ___Dyspnea on exertion
O₂ use at home? ___Yes ✔No
Chest expansion: ✔ Symmetrical ___Asymmetrical (explain: _____)
Breath sounds: ___Clear ___Crackles ___Rhonchi ✔ Wheezing Location _bilat upper lobe, inspiratory_
Cough: None ✔ Nonproductive ___ Productive ___ Describe ____
Comments: _pulse oximetry 98% on 2 L; sleeps with 2 pillows_

GASTROINTESTINAL

Stool: ✔ Formed ___ Loose ___ Liquid ___ Mucus ___ Ostomy ___ Incontinent
Color: ✔ Brown ___ Black ___ Red tinged ___ Bloody

Diarrhea ___ Constipation ___ Abdomen: ✔ Soft ___ Rigid ✔ Nontender ___ Tender ___ (Location)
Bowel Sounds ✔ Present ___ Absent ___ Hypoactive ___ Hyperactive

Obese ✔   thin ___   emaciated ___   nourished ___

*NUTRITION:
✔ Special Diet _1800 ADA_
___ Tube feeding
___ Chewing problem
___ Swallowing problems
___ Nausea/vomiting
___ Poor appetite
___ Wt. loss/gain ___ lb

* Refer to dietitian if any ✔

GENITOURINARY/ REPRODUCTIVE

Color of Urine: ✔ Yellow ___Amber ___Pink/Red tinged ___Brown ___ Orange ___Clear ___Cloudy
___Ileo-Conduit ___Incontinent ___Catheter in place ___Frequency ___Urgency
___Difficulty in initiating stream ___Pain ___Burning ___Oliguria ___Anuria
___Dialysis   Access site: ____ Date of last dialysis: ____
Comments:____
Date of LMP _1980_   Date of last PAP _5/00_   Breast self-exam ___ Yes ✔No
Use of contraceptives: ___Yes (type ____) ___No ✔N/A
    Vaginal Discharge: ___Yes (describe ____) ✔No
    Bleeding: ___Yes (amount ____) ✔No
Pregnancies: Pregnant ___Yes ___Weeks gravida ___ Para ___ ✔No
Date of last Prostate Exam ____ Testicular self-exam ___Yes ___No
Comments: ____

ACTIVITY/ MOBILITY PATTERNS

___Ambulates independently ___Full ROM ___Limited ROM (explain: ____)
✔ Ambulates with assistance (explain:____) ✔cane ___walker ___crutches
___Gait steady/unsteady ___Mobility in bed (ability to turn self) ____
Musculoskeletal ___ Pain___Weakness___ Contractures___ Joint swelling
___ Paralysis___ Deformity___ Joint stiffness___ Cast___ Amputation
Describe: ____
Comments: ____

REST/ SLEEP PATTERNS

___ Use of sleeping aids ____ Sleeps _6_ hr/day
Comments:____

Additional assessment comment: _On arrival, diaphoretic and ⊕ hand tremors. vital signs stable. glucose 56 mg/dl._
Orange juice and lunch given to pt. 2 hr postprandial glucose 204 mg/dl. Symptoms subsided with juice. Nutritionist and di-
abetes educator consulted.   _Jill O'Brien, R.N._
MRI shows no cerebral lesions. Carotid Doppler ultrasound pending.   _B. Mayer, MD_

Integrated admission database form *(continued)*

EDUCATION/DISCHARGE SECTION
Instructions: Assessment sections must be completed within 8 hours of admission. Discharge planning and summary must be completed by day of discharge.

Patient name: _Beatrice Perry_
Record number: _554691_

EDUCATIONAL ASSESSMENT

Yes	No	
✔		Patient understands current diagnosis
✔		Family/significant other understands diagnosis
✔		Patient able to read English
✔		Patient able to write English
✔		Patient able to communicate
	✔	Patient/family understands prehospital medication/treatment regimen

Emotional Factors:

Yes	No	
✔		Patient appears to be coping*
✔		Family appears to be coping*
	✔	Any suspicion of family violence
	✔	Any suspicion of family abuse
	✔	Any suspicion of family neglect

Comment: _Diabetes teaching_

Language spoken, written, and read (other than English): _____
Interpreter services needed: ✔No ___Yes
Are there any barriers to learning (e.g., emotional, physical, cognitive)? _No_
Religious or cultural practices that may alter care or teaching needs? ___Yes ✔No Describe: _____
Is pt/family motivated to learn? ✔Yes ___No describe: _____

DISCHARGE ASSESSMENT

Living arrangements/caregiver (relationship): _Lives alone_
Type of dwelling: ___Apartment ✔House ___Nursing Home ___More than 1 floor? ✔Yes___No Describe: _____
___Boarding Home ___Other _____
Physical barriers in home: ✔No ___Yes (explain): _____
Access to follow-up medical care: ✔Yes ___No (explain): _____
Ability to carry out ADLs: ___Self-care ✔Partial assistance ___Total assistance
Needs help with: ✔Bathing ___Feeding ___Ambulation ___Other
Anticipated discharge destination: ✔Home ___Rehab. ___Nursing Home ___SNF ___Boarding Home
___Other
Currently receiving services from a community agency? ___Yes ___No
If yes, check which one ___visiting nurses ___Meals on Wheels
Concerned about returning home? ___Being alone ___Financial problems ___Homemaking ___Meal prep.
___Managing ADLs ___Other

Assessment completed by: _Jill O'Brien, R.N._ Date _2/28/01_ Time _1430_
Assessment completed by: _B. Mayer, MD_ Date _2/28/01_ Time _1445_

DISCHARGE PLANNING

Resources notified:	Name	Date	Time	Signature
Social worker				
Home care coordinator	M. Murphy, RN	2/28/01	0900	M. Murphy, RN
Other_____				

Equipment/Supplies needed: _Stair chair_
Arranged for by: _M. Murphy, RN_ Date _2/28/01_ Time _0930_
Comment: _Daughter to stay with pt at home_

DISCHARGE SUMMARY

Alterations in patterns: If yes, explain.	Yes	No	Explanation
Nutrition	✔		Adherence to ADA diet regimen
Elimination		✔	
Self-care		✔	
Skin integrity		✔	
Mobility	✔	✔	Needs help with stairs
Comfort pain		✔	
Mental status/behavior		✔	
Vision/Hearing/Speech		✔	

Discharge instructions given (specify): _Standard hosp. discharge instruction sheet_
Effects of illness on employment/lifestyle: _____
Central venous line removed: _N/A_ By whom: _____
Belongings sent with patient: ✔clothes ✔dentures ✔eyeglasses ___hearing aid ___prosthesis ___valuables
✔prescriptions ✔other _Cane_
Follow-up medical supervision to be provided by: _Dr. Schneider_
✔Patient/family instructed to call for follow-up appointment Discharge destination: _Pt's home with daughter_
Section completed by: _C. Rafferty, RN_ Date _2/28/01_ Time _1130_

from various monitors. As a nursing student, you're probably familiar with these devices in other settings, but expect to need time to adapt to integrating usage of these devices into your patient care.

Fancy formats

Narrative documentation used to be the primary means of recording data. But recently, newer formats, such as SOAP charting (subjective data, objective data, assessment data, and plan), problem-oriented charting, and flowsheets, have become more common.

Specialty assessments

Your patient's age and health status may require you to perform a more specialized examination. Specialty assessment tools include the Glasgow Coma Scale, pain rating scales, Mini-Mental Status Examination, and Dubowitz Gestational Age Assessment. The most common special assessments are those used for special populations, such as pediatric, elderly, maternal, and psychiatric patients.

You—the indispensable tool

Although standardized formats, specialty forms, and computerized data collection enhance and promote information collection and health care delivery, you—the nurse—are the primary collector of patient data. No matter what format your facility uses, data gathering and interpretation remain largely nursing responsibilities.

As a nurse, you're the ultimate—and indispensable—assessment tool. Not even the most sophisticated data collection tool or device can replace assessment by a skilled nurse.

Identifying growth and development stage

As children grow, they develop intellectually, morally, emotionally, sexually, socially, and spiritually. They learn to think abstractly and logically, use language, and explore the world around them. However, some theorists posit that growth and development don't end with childhood.

Erik H. Erikson is one of several theorists who explained how growth and development occur across the life span. As part of your assessment documentation, your instructors may ask you to identify which developmental stage your patient's growth represents. Although Erikson specifies an age range for each stage, don't be afraid to question whether your patient actually resembles a person facing the issues described. Some individuals may be mature beyond their years, while others may never have resolved the main crisis of a previous stage. Remember that you must be able to state why you believe your patient is moving through a particular stage. However, you aren't expected to be an expert in this area because you're still building your observation, listening, and communication techniques. Becoming familiar with Erikson's theory though will help you identify and better understand your patient's psychosocial needs and may be helpful in planning a teaching strategy.

Eight is enough

According to Erikson, psychosocial development occurs in eight distinct stages, which he called "the eight stages of man." During each stage, a specific conflict occurs that the person must resolve. To resolve the conflict, the person undergoes a personality change, which gives him the strength to deal with the next developmental stage. If he can't resolve a conflict at a particular stage, he'll confront it later in life.

Stage 1: Trust vs. mistrust

During the first stage, which occurs from birth to about age 1, children develop trust if their needs are met. If their needs aren't met—or are met unpredictably—they become mistrustful.

Stage 2: Autonomy vs. shame and doubt

The second stage occurs between ages 1 and 3, when children learn to control their body functions and become increasingly independent. During this stage, they prefer to do things themselves and learn autonomy largely by imitating others. If they aren't allowed to be independent or are belittled for their efforts, they develop a sense of shame and self-doubt.

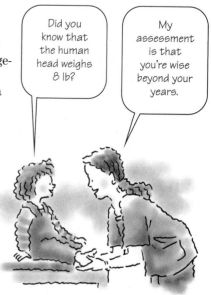

Did you know that the human head weighs 8 lb?

My assessment is that you're wise beyond your years.

Stage 3: Initiative vs. guilt

During stage 3, which occurs between ages 3 and 6, children learn about the world through play and learn to cooperate with others. They develop a conscience and learn to balance their sense of initiative against the guilt they experience for doing something against their parents' wishes. If they fail this developmental stage, as adults they may be immobilized by guilt and continue to depend unduly on others.

Stage 4: Industry vs. inferiority

During stage 4, which occurs between ages 6 and 12, children enjoy working on projects and working with others. They tend to follow rules and become competitive. Social relationships take on great importance. If unrealistic expectations (or what they perceive as unrealistic expectations) are placed on them, they may develop feelings of inferiority. However, if they develop a sense of industry, they'll feel competent to meet life's expectations.

Stage 5: Identity vs. role confusion

From ages 12 to 18, adolescents experience rapid changes in their bodies. During this stage, they're preoccupied with how they look and how others view them. While trying to meet their peers' expectations, they also try to establish their own identity. If they fail to accomplish these tasks, they can suffer role confusion. If they navigate this stage successfully, they become confident adults who feel comfortable with who they are.

Stage 6: Intimacy vs. isolation

During this stage, young adults (ages 18 through 40) seek mutually satisfying relationships, including friends and marital partners. Many of them start families. Those who negotiate this stage successfully can experience intimacy on a deep level. Those who fail to do so become isolated and distant from others. Eventually, they may withdraw socially.

Stage 7: Generativity vs. self-absorption

During middle adulthood (ages 35 to 65), work and family take on great importance. People tend to be occupied with meaningful and creative work. They strive to contribute to the betterment of society and community, to transmit cultural values through the family, and to establish a stable environment. As their children leave the home or their relationships or goals change, major life changes may occur and they struggle to find new meanings and purposes (commonly referred to as a *midlife crisis*). Failure to negotiate this stage successfully can lead to self-absorption and stagnation.

Stage 8: Integrity vs. despair

During late adulthood (ages 65 to death), people look back on their lives and accomplishments. If they have found a meaningful role in life, have a positive self-concept, and can be intimate without strain, guilt, or regret, they have a feeling of integrity. On the other hand, those who despair at their experiences and perceived failure may fear death as they struggle to find purpose in their lives.

Integrating assessment into caregiving tasks

The key to accomplishing multiple responsibilities in a short time is to view all patient care tasks as opportunities to uncover critical information. Every contact you have with a patient gives you an opportunity for assessment. Crucial information may come to light even during seemingly insignificant interactions. Answering the call light, assisting with bathing, helping with range-of-motion exercises, even making casual conversation during treatments and medication administration—these are all chances to observe the patient and gather valuable information.

Example

Suppose, for example, that you're beginning your shift assignment. One of your patients is a 45-year-old woman who was admitted for cholecystectomy. The nurse presenting the change-of-shift report notes that the patient has been demanding and has been continually pressing the call light. The patient's chart indicates that her vital signs have been stable, she has reported good pain control, and she shows no signs of postoperative complications.

Dig deeper

Instead of simply accepting the "demanding" label used by the exasperated nurse on the previous shift, you decide to investigate the patient's condition and seek more information, suspecting that the patient's behavior could signal something deeper. Instead of waiting for the patient to press the call light, you take the initiative to check on her frequently. Over the next 2 hours, the patient appears to become more relaxed.

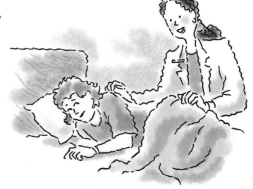

Remember that routine caregiving tasks provide an opportune time to collect valuable assessment data.

You decide to use the opportunity of morning care to spend a little extra time with the patient and assess her emotional and psychological status. As the patient washes her face and upper body, you stand quietly by her side. After a few moments, you ask her how she feels about her recent surgery and her recovery so far. She confides that she's been upset with her care in the hospital and also doesn't know how she'll manage at home. She begins to talk about all the problems she's had since the gallbladder attack just before admission. You listen carefully as the patient finishes washing, interjecting occasionally to show her that you're paying attention. As you begin massaging her back with lotion at the end of the bath, the patient tearfully reveals that her husband passed away several weeks ago—important information about the patient that you didn't previously know. During the seemingly routine chore of bathing, you have obtained information that could prove crucial to the patient's recovery and follow-up care—information that could help you to create a more appropriate care plan for this frightened, grief-stricken patient.

Data uncovered

As you can see from the previous example, taking time to assess the patient as you perform other caregiving tasks can help you to build rapport and uncover important patient information that may be crucial to your care plan.

Starting a concept map based on assessment data

In nursing school, you gain a tremendous amount of knowledge. But do you wonder how to put this theoretical knowledge into practice, especially when you have to care for more than one or two patients? Do you wonder how to start a care plan from your assessment data? Let's look at a possible scenario.

Example

You're a senior nursing student in your final rotation at a small community hospital. You're assigned to three patients on the medical-surgical unit. But before you can take vital signs on your patients, you learn you'll be receiving a pediatric patient from the ED because the pediatric unit is full. You look at your clinical instructor, hoping that she'll step in to change your assignment. Instead, she explains that the acuity level in the hospital has changed and that this will be a good opportunity for you to explore your clinical skills. Two of your other three patients are reassigned to other nurses.

The pediatric patient from the ED, John Scott, arrives within minutes. You observe that he's anxious, crying, and clinging to his mother, Christine Scott. The ED nurse gives the following report:

The patient is an 8-year-old male who has had a high fever and severe stomach pain for the last 8 hours; abdominal guarding is present. Vital signs include temperature, 101.6° F, heart rate 124 beats/minute, respiratory rate 28 breaths/minute, and blood pressure 132/80 mm Hg. Complete blood count and blood chemistry samples have been sent to the laboratory, along with a urine specimen for urinalysis. The patient is scheduled for an emergency exploratory laparoscopy within the hour to rule out a ruptured appendix.

You note that the boy's mother seems shaken and holds her child closely. Before leaving, the ED nurse takes you aside and tells you the mother is worried about the financial impact of this unexpected surgery. She hands you the patient's chart and leaves.

Don't push the panic button!

You're already running behind with your other patient. How can you possibly fulfill your nursing responsibilities to her and to your new pediatric patient? You need to admit the pediatric patient, introduce him to the hospital environment, assemble his chart, carry out the practitioner's admitting orders, verify that the necessary consents have been signed, make sure that the laboratory test results are back, and prepare the child (and his mother) for surgery. What's more, you need to perform an initial nursing assessment and then organize and document your findings before the boy goes to surgery so you can begin to develop a care plan. That's a tall order for a nursing student—or for *any* nurse. How would you handle it?

Chances are, you would feel overwhelmed, and your mind would race with frantic thoughts, such as: "Yikes! I have way too much to do and not nearly enough time to do it! So much is expected of me—and so fast. How can I meet all these demands and still make sure that my other patient is safe and receives good care?"

When asked to a panic party, turn down the invitation!

Serenity now

Remember not to panic. You're only human and can't possibly do everything at once. Before you can attend to your duties, you must attend to yourself, so take time to calm down and collect yourself. One way to do this is to stop, look, and listen. As a child, you were probably taught to stop, look, and listen before crossing a street. The same procedure can help you focus when you find yourself in a stressful patient care situation. In this case, you stop first and then analyze what you've already looked at and listened to.

Stop sign

STOP stands for:
• **S**low down—Anxiety causes the release of adrenaline, a natural stimulant. (More stimulation is the last thing you need now!)
• **T**ake some deep breaths—However many it takes to calm down.
• **O**bjectify your feelings—That is, treat them impersonally; you don't have to deny them, but you can choose to not let them control your actions.
• **P**repare a plan and proceed professionally.
After you accomplish the first three steps, the last one will be much easier. A plan gives you structure and direction and can be especially reassuring when you're feeling stressed out.

You know more than you know

Once you "stop" as described above, you'll find you feel less anxious, more in charge, and better able to think like a professional. Now, you're ready to analyze and organize the information you've already looked at and listened to—namely, the impressions you started to form from the time you met the patient and his mother and heard the ED nurse's report. That's right—you've been gathering assessment information without really being aware of it.

Let's look at what you know so far:
• The patient is 8 years old.
• He has a high fever and is in pain.
• He has just been introduced to the strange sights, sounds, smells, and people in the hospital and has just heard people talking about him rather than to him.
• He's old enough to understand what surgery is.
• He's emotionally upset, and his mother is upset as well.

As you begin your structured nursing assessment, you'll build on the developmental, emotional, physical, and social information you've already collected.

Taking time for a concept map—what a concept!

Even in a hectic situation such as this, you might quickly sketch a concept map for yourself to help you focus on what you know and what you need to know. Utilizing just the data you've been given and what you've observed, you can rough out a concept map. (See *Getting started.*)

After you've gathered the patient assessment data, you're ready to move to the next step of the nursing process—formulating nursing diagnoses. As you learned in chapter 1, creating a concept map helps you organize your thinking and see the big clinical picture.

Under construction

Getting started

Begin your concept map for the pediatric patient described in text by placing a circle in the center of the page. In that circle, include the patient's name, age, and medical diagnosis. Also note that his mother is present, and include her name.

When you have little information but you need a plan quickly, don't try to formulate nursing diagnoses for your concept map right off the bat. Instead, jot down main categories of problems as you think of them. For example, you might start by labeling a box "GI symptoms" because you don't have enough information to get a handle on which nursing diagnoses are most appropriate. Include in this box any assessment findings that you collected from your observations and the shift report. Feel free to use abbreviations in your concept map (as shown below) to save time. Also, leave the boxes open so that you can add more information as you assess the patient and get his test results. You might not even want to draw connecting lines right away, but try to visualize the interrelationships in your mind.

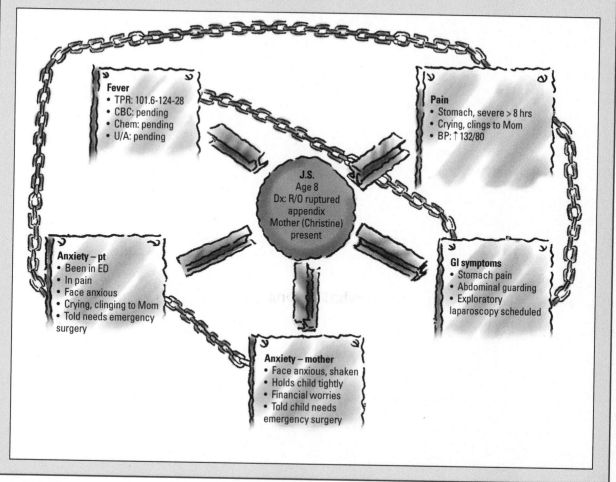

Fever
- TPR: 101.6-124-28
- CBC: pending
- Chem: pending
- U/A: pending

Pain
- Stomach, severe > 8 hrs
- Crying, clings to Mom
- BP: ↑ 132/80

J.S.
Age 8
Dx: R/O ruptured appendix
Mother (Christine) present

Anxiety – pt
- Been in ED
- In pain
- Face anxious
- Crying, clinging to Mom
- Told needs emergency surgery

GI symptoms
- Stomach pain
- Abdominal guarding
- Exploratory laparoscopy scheduled

Anxiety – mother
- Face anxious, shaken
- Holds child tightly
- Financial worries
- Told child needs emergency surgery

On the case

Case study background

Benny Hayes, a 38-year-old male, was brought to the emergency department (ED) after being involved in a boating accident. According to friends, he suffered a brief loss of consciousness at the scene. They report that he has a history of asthma. On admission, Mr. Hayes was groggy but easily aroused, scoring a 13 on the Glasgow Coma Scale. He complained of blurred vision but his pupils were equal and reactive to light and accommodation. Vital signs were stable. He presented with a 3.5 cm hematoma on his left, posterior temporal area and a deep laceration on his left forearm. A computed tomography (CT) scan with contrast of the head and X-ray of the left forearm were normal. His laceration was sutured and he was given 1 g I.V. cefazolin (Ancef) via a saline lock, as ordered. An indwelling urinary catheter was also inserted.

When you start your shift, you are assigned to Mr. Hayes. The night shift nurse reports that Mr. Hayes was admitted with a concussion. His Glasgow Coma Scale score is now 15, his speech is normal, and his pupils are equal and reactive to light and accommodation. He received 1,000 mg of acetaminophen for a headache at 6:10 a.m. His left forearm dressing is dry and intact.

As you are organizing yourself to start your care, the charge nurse tells you that Mr. Hayes' doctor has ordered removal of the indwelling urinary catheter and discontinuation of the saline lock in preparation for discharge. You decide to proceed with your morning assessment and complete the discharge paperwork before checking and carrying out these orders.

Critical thinking exercise #1

When questioned by your instructor, you give three reasons why you decided to keep the urinary catheter and saline lock in place until just before discharge. They are:

1. _____

_____

2. _____

_____

3. _____

_____

You review the chart and jot notes in concept map form, while starting to fill in the discharge sheet you'll be giving to Mr. Hayes.

Concept mapping exercise

Complete the concept map below, including the problem labels (titles for the various boxes), by integrating all of the assessment information you have so far on Mr. Hayes. Note that information from the chart review is already added for you.

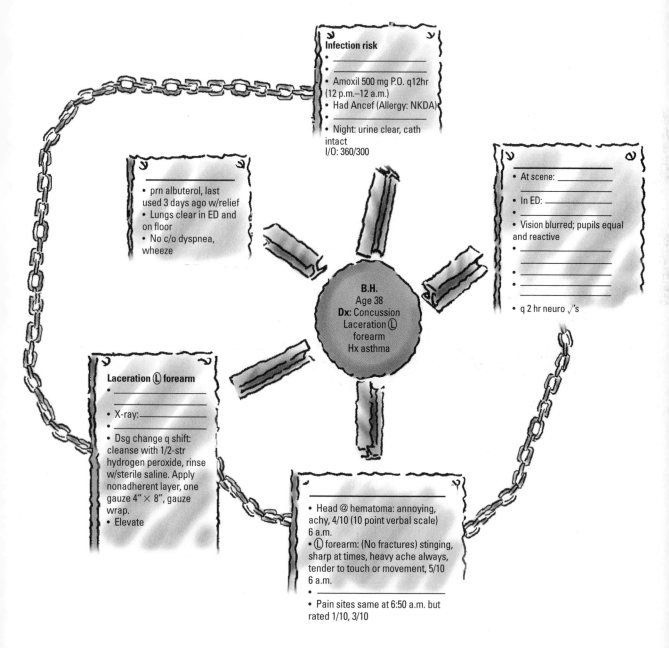

Infection risk
• _____
• Amoxil 500 mg P.O. q12hr (12 p.m.–12 a.m.)
• Had Ancef (Allergy: NKDA)
• Night: urine clear, cath intact
I/O: 360/300

• prn albuterol, last used 3 days ago w/relief
• Lungs clear in ED and on floor
• No c/o dyspnea, wheeze

• At scene: _____
• In ED: _____
• _____
• Vision blurred; pupils equal and reactive
• _____
• _____
• _____
• _____
• q 2 hr neuro √'s

B.H.
Age 38
Dx: Concussion
Laceration Ⓛ forearm
Hx asthma

Laceration Ⓛ forearm
• _____
• X-ray: _____
• _____
• Dsg change q shift: cleanse with 1/2-str hydrogen peroxide, rinse w/sterile saline. Apply nonadherent layer, one gauze 4″ × 8″, gauze wrap.
• Elevate

• Head @ hematoma: annoying, achy, 4/10 (10 point verbal scale) 6 a.m.
• Ⓛ forearm: (No fractures) stinging, sharp at times, heavy ache always, tender to touch or movement, 5/10 6 a.m.
• _____
• Pain sites same at 6:50 a.m. but rated 1/10, 3/10

You return to Mr. Hayes' room to finish your assessment and redress the laceration on his left forearm. He's sitting up in a chair and you notice that he's sleepy and his speech is slower and less clear than it had been. Nonetheless, he reports, "I feel fine. I'm just waiting for breakfast."

Critical thinking exercise #2

1. The difference in Mr. Hayes' level of consciousness (LOC) may reflect:
   a. early morning hunger.
   b. beginning infection from the indwelling urinary catheter or arm wound.
   c. an increase in intracranial pressure (ICP).
   d. a normal variant in some individuals.
2. Your first action after seeing the change in Mr. Hayes is to:
   a. call the I.V. team to obtain a blood sample to send for a chemistry profile and complete blood count, while you obtain a urine sample for urinalysis with culture and sensitivity.
   b. take his vital signs; measure his pupils; check the remainder of his neurologic signs; and assist him into bed with the rails up.
   c. put up the bed rails, give him his call bell, tell him to stay in bed, and then leave to find his primary nurse or your instructor to ask for assistance.
   d. apply oxygen and then call the practitioner immediately and request a repeat CT of the brain or magnetic resonance imaging of the brain because of a probable subdural hematoma.

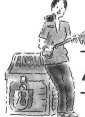

Answer key

Critical thinking exercise #1

1. If Mr. Hayes' condition suddenly changed before discharge, an I.V. line might be needed for new medications.
2. If an untoward event occurs, the indwelling urinary catheter will be necessary to assess the patient's fluid balance.
3. You're responsible for fully assessing the patient so you can complete your portion of the discharge plan.

Concept mapping exercise

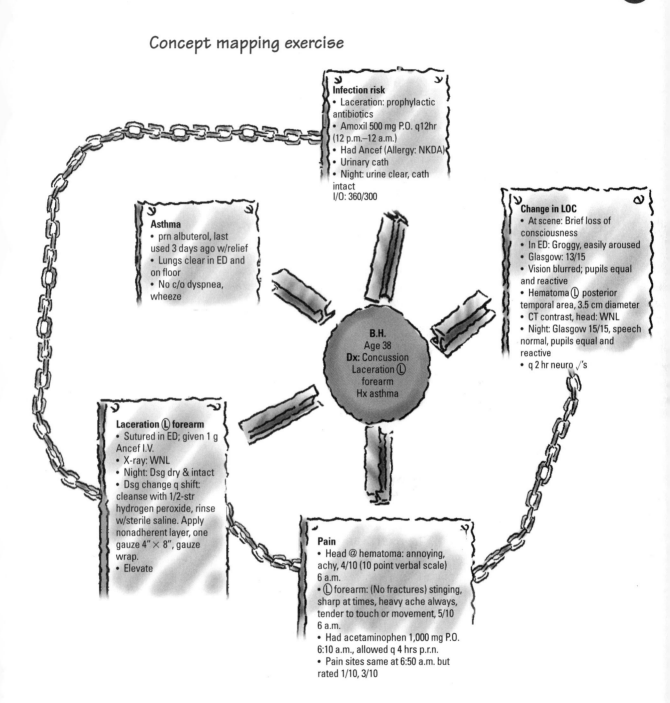

Infection risk
- Laceration: prophylactic antibiotics
- Amoxil 500 mg P.O. q12hr (12 p.m.–12 a.m.)
- Had Ancef (Allergy: NKDA)
- Urinary cath
- Night: urine clear, cath intact
I/O: 360/300

Asthma
- prn albuterol, last used 3 days ago w/relief
- Lungs clear in ED and on floor
- No c/o dyspnea, wheeze

Change in LOC
- At scene: Brief loss of consciousness
- In ED: Groggy, easily aroused
- Glasgow: 13/15
- Vision blurred; pupils equal and reactive
- Hematoma Ⓛ posterior temporal area, 3.5 cm diameter
- CT contrast, head: WNL
- Night: Glasgow 15/15, speech normal, pupils equal and reactive
- q 2 hr neuro √'s

B.H.
Age 38
Dx: Concussion
Laceration Ⓛ
forearm
Hx asthma

Laceration Ⓛ forearm
- Sutured in ED; given 1 g Ancef I.V.
- X-ray: WNL
- Night: Dsg dry & intact
- Dsg change q shift: cleanse with 1/2-str hydrogen peroxide, rinse w/sterile saline. Apply nonadherent layer, one gauze 4" × 8", gauze wrap.
- Elevate

Pain
- Head @ hematoma: annoying, achy, 4/10 (10 point verbal scale) 6 a.m.
- Ⓛ forearm: (No fractures) stinging, sharp at times, heavy ache always, tender to touch or movement, 5/10 6 a.m.
- Had acetaminophen 1,000 mg P.O. 6:10 a.m., allowed q 4 hrs p.r.n.
- Pain sites same at 6:50 a.m. but rated 1/10, 3/10

Critical thinking exercise #2

1. C. A change in LOC is an early indicator of increased ICP. Hunger and early infection don't produce this sign. A subtle change in LOC is suspicious and may be the only early sign of increased ICP in a patient with a head injury. Pupillary changes are a later sign of increased ICP.

2. B. Because Mr. Hayes isn't in acute distress, your first action would be to assist him to a safer position in case of further deterioration; then you would complete your neurologic check and vital signs assessment so you can give objective, useful information to the primary nurse or your instructor. Ordering laboratory work is out of the scope of practice of the nurse. Making the patient safe is only a portion of your responsibility when a patient's status changes; a focused assessment of the new findings must also be completed unless the change is severe and beyond your skill level. There's no indication in the data given that the patient is in respiratory distress and may need immediate oxygen therapy. Independently calling a practitioner for orders is outside the scope of practice for a student.

Nursing diagnosis

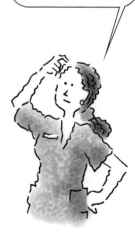

Just the facts

In this chapter, you'll learn:

♦ parts of a nursing diagnosis

♦ types of nursing diagnoses

♦ tips for identifying nursing diagnoses from concept map data.

A look at nursing diagnosis

Nursing diagnosis is the second step of the nursing process. After you've assessed the patient and clustered the findings into related areas, you must analyze these clusters to identify the patient problems that nursing care can address. Next, you'll create specific labels—nursing diagnoses—for each of your patient's problems.

A definition for the diagnosis

NANDA International (also called NANDA-I or NANDA, and formerly known as the North American Nursing Diagnosis Association) defines a nursing diagnosis as a "clinical judgment about an individual, family, or community response to actual or potential health problems or life processes which provides the basis for definitive therapy toward achievement of outcomes for which a nurse is accountable."

So what does this really mean? Let's break down this definition into digestible parts:

• A health problem is a circumstance such as illness, injury, or surgery or a lack of knowledge about a health issue. Examples of life processes include divorce, pregnancy, or the death of a loved one.

• The problem must be responsive to evidence-based, clearly outlined interventions.

Confused by NANDA? You're not alone. I need a dictionary just to understand NANDA's definition of a nursing diagnosis.

- The nursing diagnosis must reflect a problem for which the nurse:
  - is legally permitted to intervene independently
  - can be held accountable for the outcomes.

Gimme three steps, mister

To formulate nursing diagnoses, follow these three steps:

1. Identify the patient's problems—using a concept map, if necessary.

2. Write a nursing diagnosis for each problem.

3. Validate the diagnosis.

Suppose your patient reports shortness of breath while walking short distances; your assessment reveals nasal flaring, a rapid respiratory rate, and pursed-lip breathing. When clustering these data, you would see that these findings suggest a respiratory problem. Based on this, you would formulate an appropriate nursing diagnosis. Usually, your clustered data will lead you to establish several nursing diagnoses for each patient. You'll then arrange these diagnoses based on priority to ensure that you address the most crucial problems first.

Can't do without critical thinking

You'll need all your critical thinking skills to determine which nursing diagnoses are appropriate and to write diagnostic statements correctly. For example, understanding anatomy and physiology of the respiratory system and the way in which various lung disorders can alter respiratory function is critical to choosing between the nursing diagnoses *Impaired gas exchange*, *Ineffective airway clearance*, and *Ineffective breathing pattern*. If you select an inappropriate diagnosis, you're likely to choose ineffective nursing interventions, and your care plan will not only reflect your lack of understanding but will also fail to help the patient.

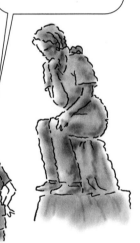

Do you like my new work? I call her the "Critical thinker." She's a favorite among nursing instructors.

Parts of a nursing diagnosis

A nursing diagnosis is commonly referred to as a *diagnostic statement* because its format includes all the information that a nurse would need to quickly understand the factors affecting a particular patient and the specific symptoms of his problem. An experienced nurse who's pressed for time could, therefore, provide appropriate care for the patient without even reading the expected outcomes and interventions listed on the care plan.

Nursing diagnoses can have three parts:

The first part is simply a **label**—for instance, *Readiness for enhanced parenting*. It describes an actual or potential patient problem that nursing care can influence. This part is usually written in NANDA-approved terminology.

Part two is the **etiology,** the related factors that precede, contribute to, or are associated with the patient's problem. Examples of related factors include diseases, injuries, birth defects, inherited patterns, signs or symptoms, medical procedures, psychosocial factors, developmental phases, lifestyle, and situational or environmental factors. In the diagnosis, the etiology should be preceded by the words "related to," as in *Self-care deficit (bathing/hygiene) related to weakness.*

The third part of a nursing diagnosis is a list of the **signs and symptoms** that support the diagnosis. This part is preceded by the phrase "as evidenced by." For example, a three-part diagnosis for a psychiatric patient might read *Ineffective role performance (work) related to depression as evidenced by decreased concentration, increased daily sleep pattern, and frequent crying while awake.*

Memory jogger

When thinking about the three parts of a nursing diagnosis, remember that **LESS** is more. A nursing diagnosis that includes all three parts, (Label, Etiology, Signs, and Symptoms) provides the most information about the patient's condition.

When to use which parts

You may notice that nursing textbooks, journals, and research papers sometimes refer to only one part of a nursing diagnosis (the diagnostic label) when defining patient problems. In some cases, the other two parts may be too specific for the discussion and are, therefore, unnecessary. In other cases, however, more detail is required and the diagnosis may include the etiology as well.

The care plans that you write for school or in practice must include at least the first two parts of the diagnostic statement. Furthermore, if you're writing about a patient's existing problem, all three parts of the statement would be necessary for another nurse to understand the patient's situation. If the patient has the potential to develop a particular problem, but no current signs and symptoms, then the correctly written nursing diagnosis would contain just the first two parts of a diagnostic statement.

Types of nursing diagnoses

NANDA-I recognizes four types of nursing diagnoses:
- actual
- risk
- syndrome
- wellness.

Actual diagnosis

An actual nursing diagnosis describes an existing problem—a human response (individual, family, or community) to a health condition or life process that's validated by the presence of major defining signs and symptoms that cluster in patterns.

Everything's included

All three parts of a diagnostic statement are required for this type of diagnosis because:
- a label for the response or problem can be readily identified: *Ineffective infant feeding pattern*...
- the etiology can be specified: *...related to cleft palate*...

Under construction

Adding evidence to the diagnosis

Writing a three-part nursing diagnosis is easy if you take it step by step. After writing the diagnostic label and the "related to" portion of the nursing diagnosis, add defining characteristics—assessment findings that support the diagnostic label you've chosen. Precede these findings with the words "as evidenced by." Defining characteristics can be either subjective (such as the patient statement "I feel dizzy") or objective (such as vital signs or physical findings).

For example
For an otherwise healthy patient with an open arm fracture, you collect the following assessment findings:
- vital signs—temperature 98.9° F, pulse 104 beats/minute, respirations 20 breaths/minute, and blood pressure 124/76 mm Hg
- displacement of the humerus of the left arm, 6" above the elbow
- ragged-edged wound at the site of the injury with localized bruising, swelling, and sanguineous oozing
- displaced fracture of the left humerus on X-ray
- facial grimacing and tearfulness
- pain rating of 3 on a 0-to-10 scale
- constant twitching and movement of the legs
- tight gripping of the side rail by the right hand
- patient statement, "I'm afraid of being put under for surgery. My aunt just died that way" (when told by the orthopedic surgeon that open reduction and internal fixation of the fracture is the best treatment for this injury).

   Given the patient's statement regarding surgery, one of the nursing diagnoses you should choose is *Anxiety;* you add the statement *related to fear of anesthesia.* Then you should add the statement "as evidenced by" and choose only those assessment findings most pertinent to this particular diagnosis. Your list should include enough information to validate your choice of diagnosis but need not include every large and small piece of evidence you collected. In this example, you would complete your three-part diagnosis with *as evidenced by muscle twitching and tension and patient statement regarding anesthesia for surgery.*

• the patient exhibits qualifiable or quantifiable signs and symptoms of the response: ...*as evidenced by the inability to form a mouth seal and abdominal distention from swallowed air.* (See *Adding evidence to the diagnosis.*)

Risk diagnosis

A risk diagnosis describes a potential problem that the patient is at risk for developing. This type of diagnosis must:
• describe a problem or situation that could be prevented with proper planning and implementation of appropriate interventions
• be supported by risk factors (assessment findings) that make the patient more vulnerable to the particular problem.

Risky business

The diagnostic label for a risk diagnosis always begins with the words *Risk for.* In addition, these diagnoses always contain only the first two parts of a diagnostic statement. Because the patient is just at risk for the problem, no signs and symptoms of the diagnosis are present (and therefore, you can't include an "as evidenced by" statement); you're simply developing a plan to prevent the problem from occurring. Say, for example, your patient has a fractured femur, is restricted to bed rest, and is obese. Based on these assessment findings, you might formulate a nursing diagnosis of *Risk for injury (thrombolytic event or blood clot) related to obesity, decreased mobility, and bone fracture.*

Although the list of NANDA-approved diagnoses includes several risk diagnoses, you may also occasionally need to restate an actual diagnosis as a risk diagnosis if no other label appears appropriate.

> Risk diagnoses are easy to identify; they begin with the words "Risk for." Now that's risky business!

Syndrome diagnosis

A syndrome diagnosis is a NANDA-I label specifically designed to serve as a shortcut in special diagnostic situations. A syndrome itself represents a pattern of signs and symptoms that, when found together, form a distinct clinical disorder. In medicine, many such syndromes have been identified—for example, Cushing's syndrome, acquired immunodeficiency syndrome, and fetal alcohol syndrome. In nursing, a syndrome diagnosis is used when a cluster of assessment findings or nursing diagnoses occur together, showing a specific clinical pattern. Syndrome diagnoses can be actual or risk diagnoses.

Six degrees of syndrome

Syndrome nursing diagnoses include a label, an etiology, and a group of signs and symptoms or nursing diagnoses. They always contain the word "syndrome" in the label. NANDA-I has approved six syndrome diagnoses:

- disuse syndrome
- impaired environmental interpretation syndrome
- posttrauma syndrome
- relocation stress syndrome
- rape-trauma syndrome
- sudden infant death syndrome.

For example...

An individual with a nursing diagnosis of *Rape-trauma syndrome* might appropriately be given multiple nursing diagnoses, such as *Acute confusion, Acute pain, Anxiety, Disturbed body image, Imbalanced nutrition: Less than body requirements, Insomnia, Powerlessness,* and *Sexual dysfunction.* However, a syndrome diagnosis can be used instead to provide a concise statement about the correlation among these factors and the rape event.

Wellness diagnosis

A wellness diagnosis describes a patient's response to a level of wellness. Typically, these diagnoses are used for patients who are already healthy but want to maintain or improve their wellness levels. These diagnoses are more commonly seen in clinics and other outpatient health care settings but can be used in any setting.

> Even healthy people can be assigned nursing diagnoses. These diagnoses are called *wellness diagnoses.*

For example...

Suppose a 57-year-old male patient of normal height and weight with no history of medical problems wants to optimize his wellness by improving his diet and starting an exercise regimen. An appropriate wellness diagnosis might be *Health-seeking behaviors related to lack of knowledge about a regular exercise program.* Supporting data would include an existing wellness level and an expressed desire for optimal fitness and enhanced wellness.

Creating nursing diagnoses from a concept map

If you used a concept map to plot out your patient's assessment data, as described in chapter 2, you can then use that map to help you define the best nursing diagnoses for your patient.

Example

As an example, let's expand on the case scenario used in chapter 2 (page 56). You've settled the child and his mother into a hospital room and oriented them to the call bell system and telephone usage. The patient's and his mother's responses to your questions help you realize that they don't know what's involved in getting ready for surgery, what to expect after the surgery, or how long the surgery might last. The child is focused on his discomfort and points to the face labeled 8 on a 10-point faces pain rating card. He lies in the bed holding his abdomen, occasionally moaning, and complains of increasing nausea and head pounding. His skin is hot and dry, his color is pale, and he won't let you touch or listen to his abdomen. He hasn't experienced vomiting or diarrhea so far, and his last bowel movement was yesterday. His blood pressure is 126/74 mm Hg, temperature 102.4° F, pulse 120 beats/minute, and respirations 28 breaths/minute. His lungs are clear and all his peripheral pulses are intact.

Per the surgeon's orders, you initiate an I.V. line and start infusing dextrose 5% in normal saline solution. As you work, you explain to the patient and mother what you're doing and why. You also explain that the surgeon wants the patient to have a computed tomography (CT) scan of the abdomen before the procedure. You explain as simply as possible what a CT scan is. You also explain that the surgeon hasn't approved any pain medication because of the impending surgery (pain medication can mask important symptoms). When the patient is transported to the CT scan department, you provide more information to the mother on the surgical process and care after the procedure. The pharmacy sends up the ordered dose of I.V. antibiotics preoperatively and you verify with the mother that the child has no known drug or latex allergies. You've already informed the surgeon of the mother's concerns about finances and obtained a referral for the social worker to visit. Per the mother's wishes, you've also notified the chaplain that she would like a visit as soon as possible.

With the above data in hand, you update your concept map, including the laboratory results that have returned. (See *Concept mapping for diagnosis*, page 68.)

Concept mapping for diagnosis

Now that you have more information, you can update your concept map by adding all the assessment data you've collected (as shown here in color) or just adding a few reminders based on the health assessment form you completed for admission.

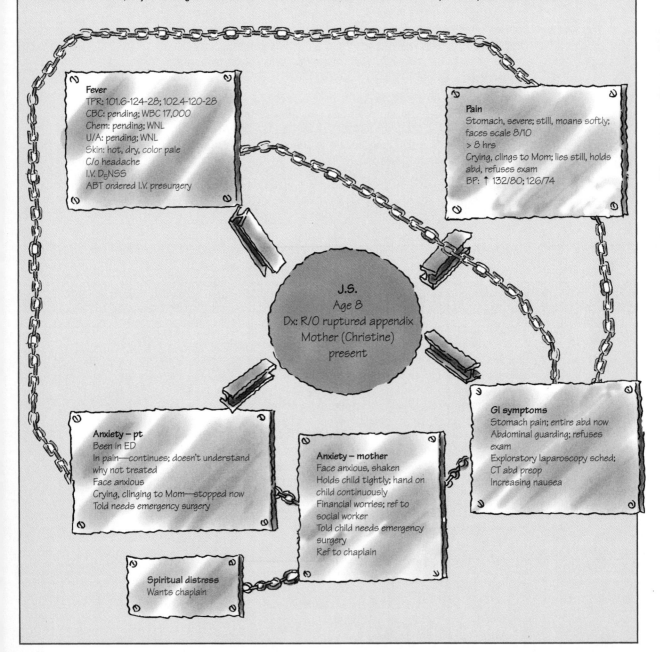

Fever
TPR: 101.6-124-28; 102.4-120-28
CBC: pending; WBC 17,000
Chem: pending; WNL
U/A: pending; WNL
Skin: hot, dry, color pale
C/o headache
I.V. D_5NSS
ABT ordered I.V. presurgery

Pain
Stomach, severe; still, moans softly;
faces scale 8/10
> 8 hrs
Crying, clings to Mom; lies still, holds
abd, refuses exam
BP: ↑ 132/80; 126/74

J.S.
Age 8
Dx: R/O ruptured appendix
Mother (Christine)
present

Anxiety – pt
Been in ED
In pain—continues; doesn't understand
why not treated
Face anxious
Crying, clinging to Mom—stopped now
Told needs emergency surgery

Anxiety – mother
Face anxious, shaken
Holds child tightly; hand on
child continuously
Financial worries; ref to
social worker
Told child needs emergency
surgery
Ref to chaplain

GI symptoms
Stomach pain; entire abd now
Abdominal guarding; refuses
exam
Exploratory laparoscopy sched;
CT abd preop
Increasing nausea

Spiritual distress
Wants chaplain

Creating a problem list

When you develop a nursing diagnosis, you're translating the patient's history data, physical findings, and laboratory data into a statement about his clinical status, responses to treatment, and nursing care needs. A good way to start is to use the assessment information you've gathered to develop a problem list, which describes the patient's problems or needs. To help generate the list, you might want to use a conceptual model, such as Gordon's functional health patterns or a concept map.

Problem child

In the problem list, identify your patient's problems and needs with simple phrases, such as "high fever" or "GI distress." Then look at the assessment data categories, such as activity-exercise pattern or health maintenance pattern. For each category, determine if your patient is having a problem or is at risk for developing one. Then formulate a tentative nursing diagnosis for each problem or potential problem. (See *Problems, problems list*.)

Problems, problems list

Once all of your assessment data are updated on your concept map, you can analyze these data to create a problem list. Find a corner on the map and list the problems you've noted. Then begin to rough out the nursing diagnoses you believe might match those problems. For example, a problem list for the patient concept map at left might include the following problems and potential diagnoses.

PROBLEMS
• Fever, ↑ WBCs: Hyperthermia, Deficient fluid volume, Risk for infection
• GI sx: Ineffective protection; Risk for injury; Nausea; Ineffective tissue perfusion (gastrointestinal)
• Pain: Acute pain
• Anxiety, mother: Anxiety, Spiritual distress, Stress overload, Compromised family coping

Writing a diagnostic statement

As previously mentioned, the primary nursing language used in schools of nursing today, as well as in most health care facilities and agencies, is that of NANDA-I. Using NANDA-I-approved nursing diagnoses advances a standard nursing language, promotes reimbursement of medical costs, and supports electronic documentation of patient care.

NANDA-I diagnoses, definitions, related factors, and defining characteristics, as well as the taxonomy derived from them, are constantly changing to reflect newly identified needs and the latest research. NANDA-I meets every 2 years to review and revise existing nursing diagnoses and approve new ones. However, debate still continues on specific wording issues, appropriateness of certain words across cultures and nations, and whether the language is truly adequate to express the close collaboration between nurses and practitioners in managing and preventing disease complications.

Tale of the taxonomy

In 2000, NANDA-I changed its nursing diagnosis classification system from the original alphabetical listing, called Taxonomy I, to a conceptual system called Taxonomy II. The new system is based largely on Gordon's functional health patterns, but with some adjustments to reduce misclassifications and redundancies. (For more information on Gordon's functional health patterns, see page 39.)

Taxonomy II has three levels:
- domains
- classes
- nursing diagnoses.

Each domain includes several classes. For instance, the self-perception domain has three classes—self-concept, self-esteem, and body image. (See *Differentiating the domains*.) Each class, in turn, has numerous approved nursing diagnoses. The self-esteem class of the self-perception domain, for instance, has three nursing diagnoses—chronic low self-esteem, situational low self-esteem, and risk for situational low self-esteem.

As of 2007, NANDA-I has approved a total of 187 nursing diagnoses. (See *Wanted: New nursing diagnoses*, page 72.)

Dazed and confused

Some nurses have trouble writing nursing diagnoses because they find NANDA-I's terminology complex and the taxonomy confusing. Rather than listing diagnostic labels strictly alphabetically, NANDA-I lists the labels alphabetically "by diagnostic concept."

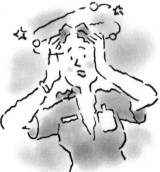

Differentiating the domains

NANDA International divides its 187 nursing diagnoses into 13 broad categories called *domains* (or *spheres of activity*):
- Health promotion
- Nutrition
- Elimination/exchange
- Activity/rest
- Perception/cognition
- Self-perception
- Role relationship
- Sexuality
- Coping/stress tolerance
- Life principles
- Safety/protection
- Comfort
- Growth/development.

Dividing the domains

Each domain has up to six subdivisions called *classes.* The domain of *Health promotion,* for instance, has two classes—health awareness and health management. On the other hand, the *Safety/protection* domain has six classes—infection, physical injury, violence, environmental hazards, defensive processes, and thermoregulation. A total of 47 classes exist among the 13 domains.

Adapted from NANDA International, *Nursing Diagnoses: Definitions and Classification, 2007-2008.* Philadelphia: NANDA International, 2007.

However, nurses who aren't familiar with the concepts contained in the list can spend time searching for a label. For example, if a patient has bowel and bladder incontinence, you might reasonably think the major concept is incontinence and go to the letter I. However, "bowel" and "urinary" (not "bladder") are the diagnostic concepts that NANDA-I links to incontinence.

Another reason that NANDA-I can be difficult to use is that not all the problems you identify on your concept map can be readily found in NANDA-I terminology. Remember the boy with GI symptoms from chapter 2? You might start looking for nursing diagnoses for this patient under the letter "G" (for gastrointestinal), figuring that diagnoses related to stomach pain would be listed there. But you find none! Now what? Here's where critical thinking can be helpful.

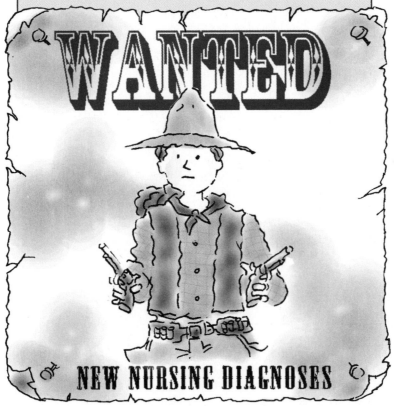

Wanted: New nursing diagnoses

NANDA International (NANDA-I) is seeking new nursing diagnoses to include in its taxonomy. Registered nurses are invited to submit new diagnoses they believe would be useful to their practice to NANDA-I's Diagnosis Development Committee (Diagnosis Review Committee). For details about submitting new diagnoses, visit *www.nlinks.org* or *www.nanda.org*.

Critically acclaimed

You apply your critical thinking skills by proposing these two questions to yourself and then answering them:

1. What type of physiology has been disrupted when severe abdominal pain and guarding and nausea are present? (*Answer:* Function of the GI tract)

2. At the simplest level, what patterns of function (NANDA-I domains) are presently most disrupted by this dysfunction within the GI tract? (*Answer:* Nutrition, activity and rest, coping and stress

tolerance, safety and protection, and comfort). (See the appendix NANDA-I nursing diagnoses by domain, pages 272 and 273.)

Stairway to labels

Next, follow these six steps to identify the NANDA-I terminology that best describes your patient's problems:

1. Look over the diagnoses listed under "Nutrition."—You decide there isn't enough evidence to support any of these diagnoses at this time.

2. Move on to the "Activity and rest" domain.—The diagnosis *Ineffective tissue perfusion (gastrointestinal)* catches your eye and you realize that this your patient's underlying problem, regardless of the exact medical cause. You write this diagnostic label down on a corner of your concept map or on a second sheet of paper.

3. Check the "Coping and stress tolerance" list.—The diagnosis *Anxiety* heads this list, and your concept map shows that the child and mother are anxious at this time, although for different reasons. You jot down this label under the previous one.

4. Scan the "Safety and protection" section.—You quickly find the diagnosis *Risk for infection,* which fits with the patient's elevated temperature, respiratory rate, and white blood cell count. You add this diagnosis to your list of labels. However, you realize you're unsure of the meanings of *Ineffective protection* and *Risk for injury,* two other diagnoses in this section.

5. Look up the NANDA-I definitions for these diagnoses and find the following definitions:

– *Ineffective protection*: "Decrease in the ability to guard self from internal or external threats such as illness or injury"

– *Risk for injury:* "At risk of injury as a result of environmental conditions interacting with the individual's adaptive and defensive resources."

Then read the related factors and defining characteristics for the protection diagnosis and the risk factors for the injury diagnosis, which help you decide that neither of these diagnoses fit the present situation.

6. Finish your search with the "Comfort" domain.—You quickly realize that this domain yields two possible diagnoses: *Acute pain* and *Nausea.* You add them to your growing list of diagnostic labels.

Whole lotta diagnoses

Now that you've chosen the diagnostic labels that best represent your assessment of the patient's problems, you must complete the diagnostic statements. This means returning to your label list and filling in the second and third parts of each statement, as appropriate. For additional tips on writing nursing diagnoses the right way, follow the guidelines outlined in *The do's and don'ts of nursing diagnoses,* pages 74 and 75.

Under construction

The do's and don'ts of nursing diagnoses

Many nurses have trouble writing nursing diagnoses using NANDA International (NANDA-I) terminology. Some find the language complex, abstract, vague, wordy, or clinically not useful. The following do's and don'ts may help you to muddle through the mass of NANDA-I's diagnoses to determine appropriate diagnoses for your patients.

Do

• Write diagnoses for problems that nurses are licensed to treat and that nursing interventions can resolve.
  – INCORRECT: *Uncontrolled blood pressure and recurrent gastroesophageal disease (daughter) related to mother's dependency on adult child for personal care as evidenced by mother's inability to be safe when alone and impaired functional capacity for personal hygiene*
  – CORRECT: *Caregiver role strain (daughter) related to mother's dependency on adult child for personal care and nurture as evidenced by mother's inability to be safe when alone and impaired functional capacity for personal hygiene*
• List the diagnostic label first and the medical cause (etiology) second.
  – INCORRECT: *Inadequate problem solving related to ineffective coping*
  – CORRECT: *Ineffective coping related to inadequate problem solving*
• Make the diagnosis clear and precise.
  – INCORRECT: *Ineffective community coping related to fear of their children catching meningitis from other school children who were close to the two girls who have meningitis as evidenced by the parents frequently keeping their children home from school and calling the practitioner to beg for antibiotics*
  – CORRECT: *Ineffective community coping related to acute meningitis outbreak as evidenced by decreased school attendance and markedly increased calls and visits to local health care providers*
• Include the diagnostic label, etiology, and signs and symptoms in all actual nursing diagnosis statements.
  – INCORRECT: *Moral distress as evidenced by patient's statements of belief in the sanctity of life from conception despite the recommendation for abortion to save the patient's life*

– CORRECT: *Moral distress related to high risk of patient's death unless fetus is aborted as evidenced by patient's statements of belief in the sanctity of life at conception*
• Include only the diagnostic label and cause in all potential (*Risk for*) nursing diagnoses.
  – INCORRECT: *Risk for infection related to chemotherapeutic immune system suppression as evidenced by probable drug nadir in 10 days*
  – CORRECT: *Risk for infection related to chemotherapeutic immune system suppression*

Don't

• Write a diagnosis that focuses on a medical problem. (Nurses are only licensed to treat nursing problems.)
  – INCORRECT: *Heart failure related to acute myocardial infarction and atrial arrhythmia*
  – CORRECT: *Decreased cardiac output related to acute myocardial infarction and atrial arrhythmia*
• Write a diagnosis that focuses on a nursing goal.
  – INCORRECT: *Promote early postoperative ambulation related to risk of prolonged immobility*
  – CORRECT: *Ineffective tissue perfusion (peripheral) related to prolonged postoperative immobility*
• Write a diagnosis that focuses on difficulty accomplishing a nursing intervention.
  – INCORRECT: *Difficulty administering tube feedings related to gastrostomy*

The do's and don'ts of nursing diagnoses *(continued)*

feeding tube insertion as evidenced by kinking of feeding tube
– CORRECT: *Imbalanced nutrition: Less than body requirements related to impaired swallowing and initiation of feeding by gastrostomy tube*
• Create a diagnosis for a treatment or diagnostic test.
– INCORRECT: *Ventilation-perfusion scan and computed tomography scan of the lungs with contrast related to risk of ineffective tissue perfusion (respiratory)*

– CORRECT: *Ineffective tissue perfusion (cardiopulmonary) related to postoperative immobility and minute thromboemboli seen on ventilation-perfusion scan*
• Say the same thing twice.
– INCORRECT: *Total urinary incontinence related to unpredictable urine loss*
– CORRECT: *Total urinary incontinence related to spinal cord injury as evidenced by inability to sense or contract the urinary sphincter*

Collaborative care

Not all nursing diagnoses can be managed solely by the nurse. To meet desired patient outcomes, some diagnoses require collaborative management by the nurse with a doctor, a nurse practitioner, a physician's assistant, a pharmacist, a dietician, a social worker, a physical therapist, a clergyperson, or another health care professional. (See *Concerns about collaborative care*, page 76.)

Elaboration on collaboration

Collaborative care is care for which:
• the practitioner is responsible for ordering definitive treatments or tests
• the nurse is responsible for implementing medical orders, acting under medically approved protocols, monitoring the patient, and taking measures to prevent complications, as needed
• the nurse may coordinate care with another health care professional under the direction of a practitioner.

Most collaborative care is tied to physiologic complications that that a nurse must monitor to detect their onset or manage changes in patient status. Examples of proposed collaborative care diagnoses might include:
• *Risk of hypovolemic shock related to blood loss*
• *Risk of postoperative complications*
• *Risk of arrhythmia related to permanent pacemaker malfunction.*

Concerns about collaborative care

Educational institutions, health care agencies, nursing professionals, and specialists on the language of nursing incorporate documentation of collaborative care within the nursing care plan in various ways.

Collaborative problem list

Lynda Juall Carpenito-Moyet, an expert on nursing diagnoses, has long advocated for care plans to include a "Collaborative Problem" category that describes physiological complications for which practitioners prescribe treatments but nurses monitor and carry out the medical and any related nursing interventions. She recommends that these problems be listed with the nursing diagnoses at the beginning of a nursing care plan and be preceded by the letters "PC," meaning "potential complication." Examples could include:
• PC: Bleeding
• PC: Pneumonia

Nursing intervention labels

Other specialists in nursing language indicate that the collaborative nature of patient care is best reflected in the nursing interventions. Thus, they list interventions as "independent" or "collaborative." Independent interventions are those that a nurse can prescribe for a human response or condition that she's legally entitled to treat.

For example, a patient who's experiencing hard stools while hospitalized may be assigned a nursing diagnosis of *Risk for constipation.* For this diagnosis, standards of nursing care would recommend such nursing interventions as providing the patient with adequate oral fluids, assisting the patient to ambulate in the hall twice per day, and teaching the patient the importance of choosing foods high in fiber. However, if the patient reports that he regularly used a stool softener at home, collaborative interventions would include reporting these findings to the practitioner and administering a daily stool softener as prescribed.

To complicate matters...

However, not all physiologic complications call for collaborative diagnoses. Suppose your patient is developing a contracture, has a stage 1 break in skin integrity, or is at risk for an infection from an external source. In this case, the nurse can initiate and implement preventive measures or order definitive treatment. Thus, the problem is considered a nursing care issue for which a nursing diagnosis is appropriate.

Create your own

NANDA-I acknowledges that not all potential nursing diagnoses, including some that relate to collaborative care, have yet been proposed or validated through their governing body. Therefore, most educational institutions allow students to include properly worded but non-NANDA-approved nursing diagnoses in their care plans. Some facilities label these diagnoses as "collaborative problems"; others handle these diagnoses in different ways.

The documentation of collaborative care concerns, as with other non-NANDA-I-approved diagnoses, remains at the discretion of the clinical or educational institution involved. This book focuses on the correct format of a nursing diagnosis and how to choose an appropriate NANDA-I nursing diagnosis. The issue of collaborative care will be discussed again in the next chapter as it relates to expected outcomes and nursing interventions. (See *Choosing a NANDA-I diagnosis*, page 78.)

Comparing nursing diagnoses and medical diagnoses

Once you become familiar with nursing diagnoses, you'll clearly see how nursing practice and medical practice differ. Both nurses and doctors identify patient problems, but they use different types of diagnoses and different treatment approaches.

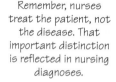

Remember, nurses treat the patient, not the disease. That important distinction is reflected in nursing diagnoses.

An interesting distinction

The main difference is that doctors are licensed to diagnose and treat a medical disease or condition, whereas nurses are licensed to diagnose and treat a patient's *response* to a disease or condition. So a nursing diagnosis describes a *response* to a disease—not the disease itself.

However, nursing diagnoses aren't limited to patients' responses to diseases. Nurses also can diagnose the need for:

- patient education
- comfort and counseling
- care until the patient is physically and emotionally capable of providing self-care.

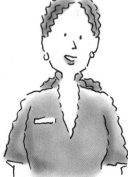

Another notable difference

Another way in which nursing diagnoses differ from medical diagnoses is that nursing diagnoses may change frequently during a patient's hospital stay or during the recovery process. As a patient progresses through the stages of illness toward problem resolution, the nursing diagnoses you formulate for him are likely to change correspondingly. (See *Adapting to changes*, pages 79 and 80.)

(Text continues on page 80.)

Teacher knows best

Choosing a NANDA-I diagnosis

What should you do if you can't easily identify a NANDA International (NANDA-I) diagnosis that applies to the patient problem you've identified? Use the algorithm below to help you.

If you have reanalyzed the data and are still convinced that no NANDA-I diagnosis is appropriate, consult with your instructor about using a non-NANDA-approved nursing diagnosis or a collaborative diagnosis.

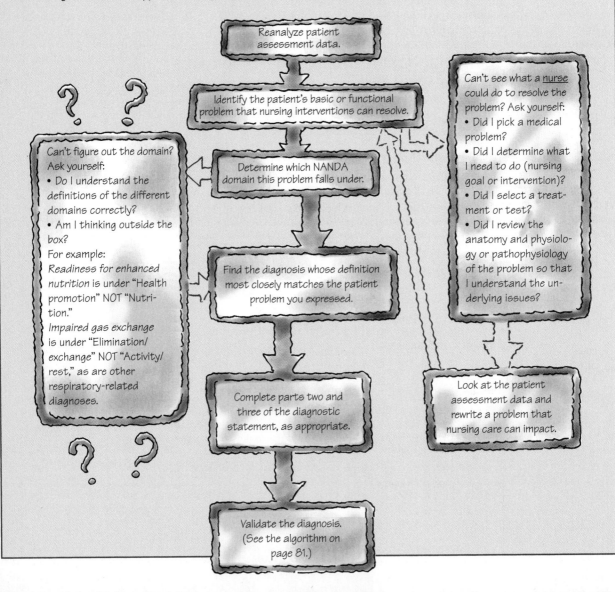

Reanalyze patient assessment data.

Identify the patient's basic or functional problem that nursing interventions can resolve.

Can't figure out the domain? Ask yourself:
• Do I understand the definitions of the different domains correctly?
• Am I thinking outside the box?
For example:
Readiness for enhanced nutrition is under "Health promotion" NOT "Nutrition."
Impaired gas exchange is under "Elimination/exchange" NOT "Activity/rest," as are other respiratory-related diagnoses.

Determine which NANDA domain this problem falls under.

Can't see what a <u>nurse</u> could do to resolve the problem? Ask yourself:
• Did I pick a medical problem?
• Did I determine what I need to do (nursing goal or intervention)?
• Did I select a treatment or test?
• Did I review the anatomy and physiology or pathophysiology of the problem so that I understand the underlying issues?

Find the diagnosis whose definition most closely matches the patient problem you expressed.

Complete parts two and three of the diagnostic statement, as appropriate.

Look at the patient assessment data and rewrite a problem that nursing care can impact.

Validate the diagnosis. (See the algorithm on page 81.)

Adapting to changes

To illustrate the variability of nursing diagnoses versus the relative stability of medical diagnoses, consider the case of J.D., a 69-year-old retired carpenter with a medical history of hypertension and hyperlipidemia. He takes olmesartan and hydrochlorothiazide (Benicar HCT) 40/25 mg and simvastatin (Zocor) 20 mg daily. He's married to 64-year-old N.D., who works 40 to 50 hours per week and also is the primary housekeeper, cook, and grocery shopper for the family. Follow his diagnoses through the course of an acute illness.

Course of the illness	Medical diagnoses	Nursing diagnoses
While his wife is at work, J.D. develops sudden, severe weakness in his right (dominant) arm and right lower lip, with milder weakness in the right leg. He calls 911 but can't relay to the responders what happened or a medical or drug history. He's confused to time and place and says anxiously, "I don't want to die." He's taken to the hospital, where a computed tomography brain scan shows no signs of cerebral hemorrhage or clotting, but his blood pressure is 192/108 mm Hg. J.D. is admitted.	Rule out: • Stroke • Hypertension • Hyperlipidemia	• *Ineffective tissue perfusion (cerebral) related to hypertension and possible stroke* • *Risk for injury related to confusion and right-sided weakness* • *Fear related to sudden body changes and risk of death*
N.D. arrives at the hospital 5 hours later but stays for only 2 hours. Within these first few hours of admission, J.D. complains to the nurse about an inability to urinate. A bladder ultrasound shows 600 ml of urine in the bladder, and the nurse inserts an indwelling urinary catheter. J.D.'s urine culture is positive for infection, and antibiotic treatment is ordered. J.D.'s weakness and confusion don't progress, and his lip drooping disappears. His blood pressure decreases to 186/96 mm Hg. J.D. still expresses fear that "this is the end."	Rule out: • Stroke • Hypertension • Hyperlipidemia • Urinary tract infection (UTI)	• *Ineffective tissue perfusion (cerebral) related to hypertension and possible stroke* • *Risk for injury related to confusion and right-sided weakness* • *Death anxiety related to sudden body changes and risk of death* • *Urinary retention related to UTI*
Gradually, all of J.D.'s neurologic symptoms disappear, except for some residual disorientation to time. J.D. verbalizes understanding that his condition is treatable. After 3 days, J.D. and N.D. are informed that discharge is imminent, and the nurse assesses their ongoing care and learning needs. N.D. has visited J.D. only briefly each day and states she has little time to learn a new diet; J.D. says he can't remember it all. J.D. is discharged from the hospital with a referral for home care services due to ongoing concerns for home safety and health maintenance and the need for more teaching regarding blood pressure management.	• Transient ischemic attack (TIA) • Hypertension • Hyperlipidemia • UTI	• *Deficient knowledge (patient): Medication regimen related to new antihypertensive and anticlotting medications* • *Deficient knowledge (patient and wife): Low-salt, low-fat diet related to new diet orders* • *Risk for injury related to possible recurrence of TIA or stroke*

(continued)

Adapting to changes *(continued)*

Course of the illness	Medical diagnoses	Nursing diagnoses
The home care nurse visits J.D. the following evening and completes an assessment. N.D. is present for the visit and expresses minimal willingness to learn about recommended dietary adjustments. She states: "I'm just too busy; I can't do it all. He needs to do more for himself and the house. He's gotten so lazy." J.D. also admits to not taking his medications regularly before the hospital admission.	• TIA • Hypertension • Hyperlipidemia	• *Deficient knowledge (patient and wife): Low-salt, low-fat diet related to new diet orders* • *Deficient knowledge (patient): Medication regimen and risk factors for stroke related to inadequate time for teaching due to patient's learning style (repetition and demonstration required)* • *Ineffective family therapeutic regimen management related to interspousal conflict over roles and skills* • *Risk for injury related to deconditioning during hospitalization, hypertension, and risk of stroke or TIA*
During the course of J.D.'s care, the home care nurse reports to the practitioner that the patient shows difficulty with short-term memory and has a Mini-Mental Status Examination score of 26 (indicative of early dementia). The practitioner orders a magnetic resonance image of the brain, which shows signs of multiple small infarctions. N.D. verbalizes more acceptance of J.D.'s caregiving needs and willingness to learn new skills when the testing shows he isn't deliberately refusing to be responsible.	• TIA • Hypertension • Hyperlipidemia • Multi-infarct dementia	• *Deficient knowledge (patient and wife): Multi-infarct dementia* • *Deficient knowledge (patient and wife): Low-salt, low-fat diet related to new diet orders* • *Impaired memory related to cerebral injury* • *Risk for injury related to deconditioning during hospitalization, hypertension, and risk for stroke or TIA*

Validating nursing diagnoses

After you have finished developing all of the patient's nursing diagnoses, you must go back and check each of the statements again to validate them. Start by determining the correctness of each diagnostic label, reviewing its definition and defining characteristics or risk factors and comparing them to the patient assessment data. Then critically analyze your information from the assessment data and your knowledge of the associated medical disorders, verifying that you accurately listed the etiology and stated the specific signs and symptoms that validate the diagnosis. This process of review and validation might help you find mistakes in interpretation of a definition or in placement of the parts of the statement. (See *Validating a diagnosis.*)

Teacher knows best

Validating a diagnosis

You've completed all your nursing diagnoses statements. What's next? Validation of the diagnoses. Follow the rest of the algorithm on your path to understanding the trick to successful nursing diagnosis.

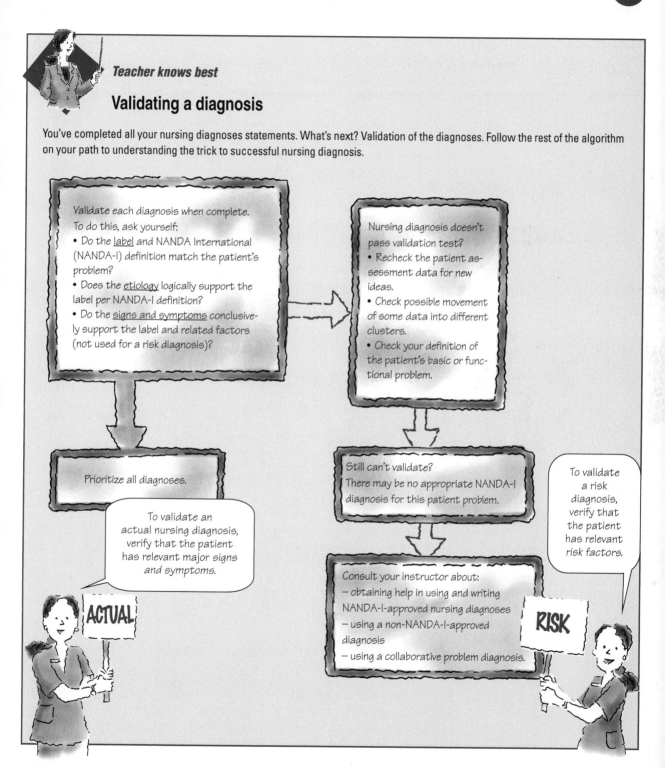

Validate each diagnosis when complete. To do this, ask yourself:
• Do the <u>label</u> and NANDA International (NANDA-I) definition match the patient's problem?
• Does the <u>etiology</u> logically support the label per NANDA-I definition?
• Do the <u>signs and symptoms</u> conclusively support the label and related factors (not used for a risk diagnosis)?

Nursing diagnosis doesn't pass validation test?
• Recheck the patient assessment data for new ideas.
• Check possible movement of some data into different clusters.
• Check your definition of the patient's basic or functional problem.

Prioritize all diagnoses.

Still can't validate?
There may be no appropriate NANDA-I diagnosis for this patient problem.

To validate an actual nursing diagnosis, verify that the patient has relevant major signs and symptoms.

To validate a risk diagnosis, verify that the patient has relevant risk factors.

Consult your instructor about:
– obtaining help in using and writing NANDA-I-approved nursing diagnoses
– using a non-NANDA-I-approved diagnosis
– using a collaborative problem diagnosis.

ACTUAL

RISK

Searching for support

If most of the patient's assessment data aren't consistent with or don't support the nursing diagnosis, you can either:
• reassess the patient for additional assessment data that *do* support the diagnosis
• revise the diagnosis so it's consistent with the assessment data.

Don't initiate the care plan until you've validated the diagnoses. If you write a care plan based on invalid nursing diagnoses, you'll waste time implementing it—and you could jeopardize your patient's well-being.

Prioritizing nursing diagnoses

Usually, you won't have time to address all—or even most—of the nursing diagnoses you've formulated for your patient. You'll need to focus on the most important ones, which means that you'll have to be able to prioritize them. Then, when you plan your care, you address the highest-priority diagnoses first.

High, low, and in between

You can prioritize diagnoses into high-, intermediate-, and low-priority:
• *High-priority* nursing diagnoses involve emergency or immediate physical care needs.
• *Intermediate-priority* diagnoses involve nonemergency needs.
• *Low-priority* diagnoses involve needs that don't directly relate to the patient's illness or prognosis.

For example, for an acute-care patient in a nonpsychiatric setting, high-priority nursing diagnoses typically relate to airway, breathing, and circulation (for example, *Decreased cardiac output related to cardiac tamponade*). Intermediate-priority diagnoses relate to problems whose resolution can impact the patient's speed or degree of recovery but aren't life-threatening (for example, *Risk for infection related to indwelling urinary catheter*). Lower-priority diagnoses commonly address anxiety, fear, self-esteem, or a preexisting chronic problem to which the patient has adapted (for example, *Insomnia related to variable shift work schedule as evidenced by sleeping during the day, awake at night since hospitalized*).

Prioritizing props

You can use the problem list you created to help you prioritize nursing diagnoses, or you can refer to Maslow's hierarchy of needs. This hierarchy classifies human needs based on the concept that physiologic needs must be met before more abstract needs can be addressed. (See *The power of Maslow's pyramid.*)

Out of time

You might need to provide a referral to the patient at discharge to help him manage ongoing recovery or long-term impairment, problems that a nurse in an acute care setting can't fully address. If your clinical experience sends you to a rehabilitation facility, skilled nursing facility, inpatient psychiatric center, or home health care agency, your care plan should address the long-term needs and concerns of the patient.

The pyramids have mystical powers. Maslow's has the power to help you prioritize nursing diagnoses.

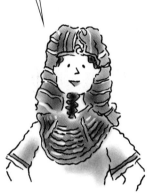

The power of Maslow's pyramid

Maslow's pyramid can help you prioritize a patient's nursing diagnoses. Physiologic needs—represented by the base of the pyramid in the diagram below—must be met first.

Self-actualization
Recognition and realization of one's potential, growth, health, and autonomy

Self-esteem
Sense of self-worth, self-respect, independence, dignity, privacy, self-reliance

Love and belonging
Affiliation, affection, intimacy, support, reassurance

Safety and security
Safety from physiologic and psychological threat, protection, continuity, stability, lack of danger

Physiologic needs
Oxygen, food, elimination, temperature control, sex, movement, rest, comfort

SELF-ACTUALIZATION
SELF-ESTEEM
LOVE AND BELONGING
SAFETY & SECURITY
PHYSIOLOGIC NEEDS

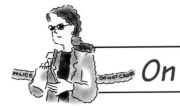

On the case

Case study background

Your patient, Harriet Zoose, has a medical diagnosis of *Acute exacerbation of ulcerative colitis.* When you obtain her health history, she tells you that she's currently experiencing painful abdominal cramps and has had very frequent bowel movements containing blood and pus for the past few days. She rates her discomfort level at a 7 on a 10-point scale. She also states she has recently had trouble sleeping and feels extremely fatigued. She says the colitis has drastically decreased her sex drive, which is causing tension within her marriage.

On physical examination, you assess:
- hypotension
- low-grade fever
- hypoactive bowel sounds
- abdominal distention and tenderness
- pallor.

When you review her diagnostic data, you note that she has a moderately elevated white blood cell count; slightly elevated blood urea nitrogen (BUN) level; decreased hemoglobin level, hematocrit, and total protein level; and a prolonged bleeding time. An upper GI series performed the previous day found scarred and stenotic bowel segments, which are obstructing the intestinal flow.

Critical thinking exercise

Together, the nursing and medical diagnoses—and the care plan overall—
should describe the complete nursing care the patient needs. For this patient,
the care plan should include nursing diagnoses that address her *response* to
her medical diagnoses. List four three-part nursing diagnoses for this patient.
(Note that there are more than four correct answers.)

1. _____

_____

_____

2. _____

_____

_____

3. _____

_____

_____

4. _____

_____

_____

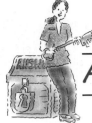

Answer key

Here are some examples of nursing diagnoses that could be appropriate for this patient:

1. *Risk for infection related to potential bowel perforation and general debilitation as evidenced by fever, abdominal distension, and hypoactive bowel sounds*

2. *Chronic pain related to abdominal cramping and distention as evidenced by pain scale rating and patient statements*

3. *Insomnia related to anxiety and uncomfortable sensations as evidenced by patient statements*

4. *Ineffective sexuality pattern related to decreased physical energy and chronic, uncomfortable physical symptoms as evidenced by decreased sexual interest per patient statements*

5. *Deficient fluid volume related to acute diarrhea and blood loss as evidenced by decreased hemoglobin level and hematocrit, increased BUN level, and decreased blood pressure*

6. *Fatigue related to decreased sleep, pain, and exacerbation of colitis as evidenced by patient statements and decreased hemoglobin level and hematocrit*

7. *Interrupted family processes related to increased symptoms of ulcerative colitis as evidenced by patient complaints of decreased libido and resultant marital tension*

Planning

Just the facts

In this chapter, you'll learn:

♦ skills for developing and writing measurable, achievable patient outcomes

♦ factors that influence behavior and contribute to patient compliance

♦ classifications of nursing interventions

♦ guidelines for developing and writing effective nursing interventions

♦ the relevance of evidenced-based practice in planning care.

Care plan components

After you establish and prioritize a patient's nursing diagnoses, you're ready to identify patient outcomes and develop a written care plan. Recall that the nursing care plan is a written plan of action designed to help you deliver quality patient care. It's based on the problems identified during the patient's admission interview and includes these three major components:
• nursing diagnoses
• expected outcomes
• nursing interventions.

One size doesn't always fit all

Care plans may be traditional (plans that are created from scratch) or standardized (preprinted plans that can be tailored to a patient's individual needs). As a student, you'll most likely use

> Writing the care plan for a patient really starts with planning achievable goals with the patient and deciding the best ways to reach them. Gathering assessment data and developing nursing diagnoses form the basis for this plan.

some form of traditional care plan format designed by your faculty until you've gained more experience in critical thinking. You may be instructed to use this care plan in conjunction with concept mapping. During your clinical rotations, you'll consult the care plan tool used by the individual facility. Keep in mind that a patient's problems and needs can change, so you'll need to review the care plan often and modify it as necessary.

Take three giant steps

Writing an initial care plan involves these three steps:

☝ reviewing the established diagnoses and assessment data if needed

✌ identifying expected patient outcomes and specific nursing interventions to attain those outcomes

🖐 documenting the nursing diagnoses, expected outcomes, and nursing interventions in a clear, consistent format.

The first step above was covered in detail in the previous chapters. It's included here as a reminder that you should know your patient's established diagnoses and current status before you begin planning his specific care needs.

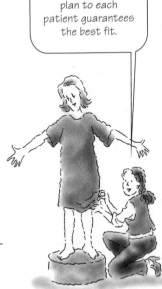

Tailoring a standardized care plan to each patient guarantees the best fit.

Identifying expected patient outcomes

During outcome identification, you must focus on determining appropriate goals, or expected outcomes, for a patient based on the nursing diagnoses you've already formulated for him. Remember, the ultimate goal of your nursing care is to help the patient reach his highest functional level with minimal risk and problems by the time of discharge. If the patient can't recover completely, your care should help him to cope physically and emotionally with his impaired or declining health.

Make sure that the outcomes in your nursing care plan focus on the patient—not on actions you must perform.

Keeping it real

With these long-range goals in mind, you need to identify realistic, measurable expected outcomes and corresponding target dates for your patient. Expected outcomes are goals the patient should reach as a result of planned nursing interventions. Sometimes, a nursing diagnosis requires more than one expected outcome.

Outcomes are always geared toward the patient's performance—not the nurse's actions. An outcome can specify an improvement in the patient's ability to function—for example, an increase in the distance he can walk—or it can specify the correction of a problem such as a reduction in pain. In either case, each outcome calls for the maximum realistic improvement for a particular patient.

Memory jogger

To remember the four necessary components of an effective outcome statement, think, "Be More Careful, Timmy":

Behavior

Measure

Conditions

Time frame.

The outcome statement

All outcomes must be patient-oriented and expressed in the form of a statement, called the *outcome statement.* For instance, a patient with a nursing diagnosis of *Impaired gas exchange related to ventilation perfusion imbalance from pulmonary embolus* might have an expected outcome of "Show decreased work of breathing and restlessness and increased oxygen saturation within 24 hours of heparin infusion initiation."

Parts of an outcome statement

An outcome statement consists of four components:

- a specific behavior that shows the patient has reached his goal

- criteria for measuring that behavior

- the conditions under which the behavior should occur

- a time frame for when the behavior should occur. (See *Understanding outcome statements,* page 90.)

Behavior

A *behavior* is generally defined as an action or response to stimulation that can be observed or heard. In terms of outcome identification, it's something (an action) you would expect to see or hear the patient do as a result of your nursing interventions.

Objectively speaking

Always begin your outcome statement with an action verb that focuses on a behavior you can objectively observe and measure. Examples of verbs that can be easily measured by sight or sound include:
- movements (for example, *ambulate, bathe, climb, give, move, perform, point, use*)

I object to subjective outcome statements. Make sure that your nursing outcomes focus on behaviors that can be objectively observed or measured.

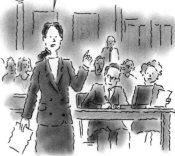

Understanding outcome statements

An outcome statement consists of four elements: behavior, measure, condition, and time frame.

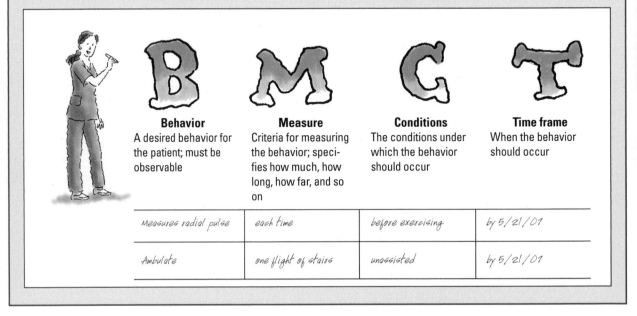

Behavior	Measure	Conditions	Time frame
A desired behavior for the patient; must be observable	Criteria for measuring the behavior; specifies how much, how long, how far, and so on	The conditions under which the behavior should occur	When the behavior should occur
Measures radial pulse	each time	before exercising	by 5/21/01
Ambulate	one flight of stairs	unassisted	by 5/21/01

- speech (for example, *describe, express, report, state, verbalize*)
- other actions (for example, *arrange, avoid, demonstrate, exhibit, identify, maintain, modify, participate, seek, set*).

Sounds subjective to me

Although it's important to consider the patient's thoughts and feelings when planning care, these can't be readily observed or measured. Avoid beginning an outcome statement with a verb that's too subjective to evaluate, such as *accept, know, appreciate,* or *understand.* After all, how can you objectively observe a patient's *appreciation?* Even when working with a psychiatric patient, you'll write outcomes based on behaviors—not the thoughts or feelings that might be influencing the behaviors. For example, instead of including the outcome "Patient will state that he feels less depressed," you might include the outcome "Patient will obtain a score of XX on the Beck Depression Scale"; this outcome is a measurable improvement in a patient's mood.

Measure

Explaining precisely what's being measured and how it's being measured helps gauge your patient's progress toward achieving his goal. It also enables you and other team members to work within consistent parameters, ensuring the systematic evaluation of nursing interventions.

Specifics, please

Make sure your outcome statement indicates the criteria needed to measure the behavior, such as:
• how much
• how long
• how far
• using what scale.

Conditions

Stipulate in the outcome statement, as necessary, the conditions under which the behavior should occur. For instance, tell when during the day the behavior should occur, how frequently it should occur, and whether the patient requires any assistance in completing the action. For example, the outcome statement, "Patient will drink 360 ml of noncaffeinated fluids on day shift, 240 ml on evening shift, and 120 ml on night shift," gives more direction to staff and sets a clearer goal for the patient than the statement "Patient will drink 720 ml of noncaffeinated fluids per day."

Don't set the bar too high

Keep in mind your patient's overall condition, ability to perform the behavior, and agreement with the proposed target. Make sure the conditions can be realistically met.

For example, you're caring for a patient who has had an acute exacerbation of moderate chronic obstructive lung disease and now requires oxygen therapy for exertion and sleep. The patient's nursing diagnoses include *Deficient knowledge (measures to maintain maximum pulmonary function) related to misconceptions about the disease process and oxygen therapy as evidenced by verbal statements regarding the disease* and *Activity intolerance related to disease process as evidenced by exertional dyspnea.* You're aware that mild but regular exercise, such as performing self-bathing and grooming activities, can help the patient maintain his residual pulmonary function, so you establish an ex-

> **Memory jogger**
>
> To differentiate objective from subjective patient behavior, think in terms of what you need to do to interpret it:
>
> Objective—Observe directly through sight or sound.
>
> Subjective—Sense what the patient is thinking or feeling.

pected outcome of "Bathe independently except for back and lower legs daily within 2 weeks." However, this outcome may not be realistic unless the patient responds to your teaching plan for *Deficient knowledge*. If the patient doesn't understand the basis for your outcome statement or doesn't agree that the goal is achievable, the expected outcome isn't realistic. In this situation, your outcome timing for the *Deficient knowledge* diagnosis must be set before the target date on the bathing outcome, and you must be prepared to adjust the bathing outcome statement depending on the patient's response to the knowledge teaching plan.

Keep time in mind. Remember to include a time frame for completing each outcome.

Time frame

Although one of your primary responsibilities as a nurse is to help your patient achieve the highest level of functioning or wellness before discharge, you need some way of monitoring his progress along the way. All patient outcomes must provide a realistic time frame for completing the desired behavior. For example, in a student care plan for a home care patient you'll be seeing once a week, you might have a new outcome statement for each visit, as you assist the patient to learn to manage his disease process. At some point in his care, you may then be able to write a longer outcome target as he gradually integrates new information and techniques into his daily routine.

The long and short of goals

Long-term goals commonly require weeks or months to achieve. Short-term goals, on the other hand, take much less time to achieve; these are typically the goals (or outcomes) you'll address in your student outcome statement. (See *Documenting long-term goals.*)

Writing outcome statements

When writing outcome statements, always start with a specific action verb that focuses on your patient's behavior. By telling how your patient should look, walk, eat, turn, cough, speak, or stand, for example, you give a clear picture of how to evaluate progress.

Choose wisely

Be careful about your verb choice, though. Such verbs as "allow," "let," and "enable" focus attention on your own and other health care team member's behavior—not the patient's behavior. In many

Documenting long-term goals

As a student, the expected outcomes you write will generally reflect short-term goals. Your instructors focus your care plans on outcomes that might be achievable by you during your clinical time with a specific patient. However, to demonstrate that you're aware of the larger issues involved in caring for a patient, you'll also probably be asked to document discharge planning. This is where you'll express the patient's long-term goals. Some of the items you may be asked to include are:
• discharge outcomes—specify the outcomes expected by the time of discharge
• learning needs—list the topics that the patient and family should demonstrate an understanding of by discharge
• referrals—explain possible referrals needed to assist the patient and his family in reaching long-term optimum health outcomes
• documentation issues—identify the results of outcome evaluation that must be documented.

To each his own

As a practicing nurse, your agency or facility may have a different system of handling short-term and long-term outcomes in its care plans. Some examples are listed here:
• Acute care settings: Factors affecting discharge planning are documented on the initial assessment. The nursing care plan lists outcomes expected by discharge. Teaching flow sheets and discharge instruction sheets are used to document learning need outcomes and patient status and medical orders plus any referrals or follow-up care upon discharge. Patients are given a copy of their discharge instructions.
• Rehabilitative, home care, long-term care settings: The nursing or interdisciplinary care plan lists short-term and long-term goals for each diagnosis and specifies dates for reevaluation of each. Discharge planning begins when the patient has been appropriately reevaluated or requests discharge. Preparations for discharge are then listed as a goal on the updated care plan, as are any continuing care needs and referrals. A discharge summary is completed on the day of discharge and a copy is given to the patient.

Find out and follow the documentation procedures at your facility.

cases, you can easily turn around outcome statements that focus on your behavior so that they focus on the patient. For example, "Medication brings chest pain relief" doesn't say anything about the patient's behavior, but "Expresses relief from chest pain within 5 minutes of receiving medication" does.

Include the nitty gritty

Also be sure to make your statements specific. For example, the statement "Understands relaxation techniques" doesn't tell you much. (How do you observe a patient's understanding?) Instead, you should write: "Practices progressive muscle relaxation techniques unassisted for 15 minutes daily by hospital day 5." This statement tells you exactly what to look for when assessing the patient's progress. Choose your words carefully and be clear and concise. (See *Tips for keeping statements concise,* page 94.)

Teacher knows best

Tips for keeping statements concise

These tips will help you write clear, precise outcome statements:
• **Avoid unnecessary words.** For example, with many documentation formats, you won't need to include the phrase "The patient will…" with each expected outcome statement. In most cases, it's obvious that you're talking about the patient. However, you'll have to specify which person the goals refer to when family, friends, or others are involved.
• **Use accepted abbreviations.** Refer to the Joint Commission on Accreditation of Health Care Organization's and your facility's list of approved abbreviations. If your facility's list describes patient stays in day-long intervals, use abbreviations such as "HD1" for hospital day 1 or "POD 2" for postoperative day 2.
• **Use a standardized list of patient outcomes,** such as the Nursing Outcomes Classification or the classification system used in your facility.

Although your outcome statements should be detailed, try to keep them clear and concise.

For your consideration

When writing outcome statements, consider the patient's medical orders. The outcome statements you write shouldn't ignore or contradict those medical orders. For example, before including the outcome statement, "Ambulate 10′ unassisted twice per day by postoperative day 3," make sure that the medical orders don't call for more restricted activity.

Also, adapt the outcome to the specific circumstances. Consider such health-related factors as the patient's coping ability, age, education, cultural influences, family support, living conditions, socioeconomic status, and anticipated length of stay. Also consider the health care setting. For example, the outcome statement, "Ambulate outdoors with assistance for 20 minutes t.i.d. by admission day 5," might be unrealistic in a facility located within a large city. (See *Factors affecting health.*)

Patient participation

One way to help ensure the effectiveness of outcome statements is to encourage the patient to participate in formulating them. A patient who helps write his outcome statements is more motivated to achieve his goals. His input, along with family member input, can also help you set realistic goals. (See *Eliciting the patient's help* and *How to obtain better patient compliance*, page 96.)

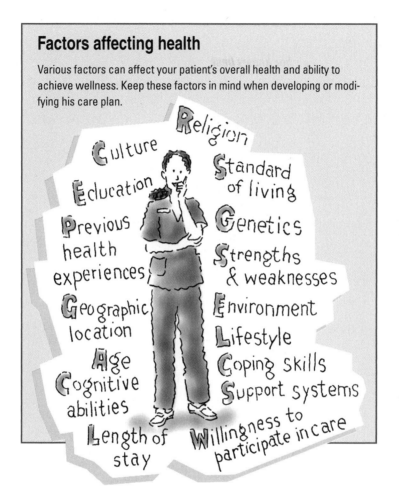

Factors affecting health

Various factors can affect your patient's overall health and ability to achieve wellness. Keep these factors in mind when developing or modifying his care plan.

Religion

Culture

Education

Standard of living

Previous health experiences

Genetics

Strengths & weaknesses

Geographic location

Environment

Lifestyle

Age

Coping skills

Cognitive abilities

Support systems

Length of stay

Willingness to participate in care

Up for a challenge?

Not all outcome statements will be as straightforward to formulate as the examples previously presented. In such cases, remembering the four components and identifying each component separately can help you formulate outcome statements. (See *Finding the right words in difficult situations,* pages 97 and 98.)

Nursing Outcomes Classification

As described in chapter 1, the Nursing Outcomes Classification (NOC) is a nursing-sensitive, standardized categorization of patient outcomes that helps nurses evaluate the effects of nursing in-

Eliciting the patient's help

Discussing the care plan with the patient and keeping him informed about his progress and needed changes can be mutually beneficial. The patient remains informed and actively involved in health care decisions, and you elicit his compliance with achieving the outcomes stipulated in the care plan. Remember to keep the following points in mind:
• Discuss the care plan with the patient, and keep him informed whenever the plan changes.
• Assess the patient's knowledge about his condition or problem.
• Explain procedures and review laboratory findings.
• Respect the patient's wishes in the decision-making process.
• Begin discussing discharge plans at the earliest appropriate time, keeping the patient apprised of necessary changes to the plan.
• Seek the patient's permission to discuss his progress and needs with his family, particularly when planning ahead toward discharge.

Weighing the evidence

How to obtain better patient compliance

In a 2004 article in the *Journal of Nursing Care Quality*, authors Maramba, Richards, Myers, and Larrabee reported their literature review research on the discharge planning process. One of the components investigated was patient satisfaction with the care provided. The authors stated that, "Two studies identified patient and family understanding of the patient's condition, feeling prepared to manage care after discharge, and being involved in decisions related to discharge planning as predictors of patient satisfaction." Other research has shown that when patients are more satisfied with their care, they're more likely to follow the care plan upon discharge.

terventions. Experience has shown, however, that the outcomes listed can be useful for other disciplines as well.

Just so we understand each other...

In order to correlate patient outcomes with specific interventions and evaluate their effectiveness in a way that's meaningful and useful, health care providers must agree on standardized definitions of the words used when talking about patient care. Such standardization serves four main purposes:
• It ensures consistent measurement and comparison of patient outcomes.
• It helps validate the effectiveness of nursing care as a component of quality, cost-effective health care.
• It further legitimizes the profession of nursing in the health care arena.
• It aids in adapting nursing care planning into the electronic health system database.

The creators of NOC have done extensive research with practicing nurses and nurse-educators in various settings to determine which words nurses regularly use in discussing the outcomes of their patient care and which tasks they perform to impact these outcomes. NOC research is ongoing to validate each outcome and indicator as well as to add new outcomes.

Finding the right words in difficult situations

Some of the most difficult nursing diagnoses to work with are those that reflect the patient's perceptions and feelings and those that refer to normal human processes such as birth. Let's look at and work through two examples.

Example diagnosis 1

In some ways, the diagnosis *Risk for disorganized infant behavior related to potential intrapartum complications* appears to have a simple outcome: the fetus will be delivered without experiencing any alteration in normal fetal signs indicative of intrapartal complications resulting in disorganized infant behavior. But how do you word the behavior, measure, condition, and time frame in the outcome statement for this generalized outcome?

One step at a time

Here are four steps for constructing an outcome statement for this diagnosis:

• Consider what actual fetal signs you can measure while the infant is in the process of being delivered (the mother is in labor). Examples might include fetal heart rate, variations in electronic fetal monitoring patterns, the presence of meconium staining of the amniotic fluid when the sac has broken, and fetal position or presenting part. Then think of an action verb to describe the **behavior** (sign) you wish to see. Examples might include "Maintain fetal heart rate" or "Detect meconium staining of the amniotic fluid."

• Determine the limits for the behavior—in other words, the way in which you would **measure** the success or failure of your outcome. For "Maintain fetal heart rate," you would want to specify the normal fetal heart rate range during labor, which is 120 to 160 beats/minute. For "Detect meconium staining of amniotic fluid," you would expect the amniotic fluid to be clear or have a yellow or green tinge upon rupture of the amniotic sac, not marked by the dark green color of meconium. If staining were present, the infant would be at risk for aspiration of meconium during the intrapartum period.

• Outline the **conditions** under which you would expect to find the two behaviors listed above. In normal labor, the fetal heart rate would remain within the cited limits throughout the delivery process. But detection of the color of the amniotic fluid (the indicator for the risk of aspiration of meconium) must be stated more specifically, by saying, for example,

"immediately," "within 5 minutes," "within 2 hours," or whatever time you believe is realistic considering the situation.

• Last, state the **time frame** within which you would expect to accomplish the stated outcomes. In this situation, the time frame can be the period ending with the birth of the infant or, for the amniotic fluid, the time after the amniotic sac has broken.

Putting it together

For this diagnosis, you could make two clear outcome statements using the guidelines above:

• Maintain fetal heart rate within 120 to 160 beats/minute throughout the intrapartal period until birth.

• Detect meconium staining of the amniotic fluid by presence of dark-green color of the fluid within 5 minutes of rupture of the amniotic sac.

As you can probably see, several other possibilities for specific outcome statements exist for this diagnosis. As a student, you would choose only those for which you could be accountable during your clinical time with the patient.

Example diagnosis 2

Let's look at another example with a different type of diagnosis: *Ineffective denial related to new diagnosis of pulmonary hypertension (PH) as evidenced by patient statements, "I feel better already. You just let me go home, and I'll get back to work in no time" and "I think I was just working too much overtime and got exhausted. I just needed a break."* The first tendency would be to write the outcome statement: "Patient will accept his new diagnosis of PH by discharge." However, because "accept" is a subjective verb, this outcome is hard to measure. Taking one component at a time, let's see how to word a reasonable outcome for this patient:

• Objective desired **behaviors** might include "Describes PH as the source of changes in functional capacity," "Expresses interest in learning more about the disease," "States understanding of the chronic and progressive nature of the disease," and "Questions staff about how the disease may affect his ability to return to work after hospital discharge."

(continued)

Finding the right words in difficult situations (continued)

• Let's assume that your interactions with the patient have led you to choose "Describes PH as the source of changes in functional capacity" as an attainable behavioral outcome. Possible **measurement** of that behavior might be "by citing PH, not overwork or exhaustion, as the source of symptoms."

• The **conditions** under which you might reasonably expect the patient to demonstrate this desired behavior might be "daily, when queried by nurse."
• "Within 3 days of diagnosis" is a clear **time frame** for the expected behavior, although a specific date would be more helpful to other staff nurses.

What NOC is not

Perhaps the most confusing thing about using NOC is understanding that a NOC outcome *isn't* the same as a nursing goal or expected outcome. By definition, it's an individual patient's state or behavior, including perceptions or subjective states. In fact, NOC outcomes are deliberately designed to be variable, not goal-specific. What does this mean? It means that a NOC outcome:

• defines a patient's state at a specific time, which can represent an improvement or a decline from that patient's state at an earlier assessment
• becomes an "outcome" only if it's assessed after a nursing intervention (thus, a patient's mobility status on an admission assessment is information, not an outcome)
• is measured along a continuum from negative to positive
• has an associated group of specific state, behavior, or perception descriptions (called *indicators*) that give examples of the various components of the outcome
• can apply to any discipline if they use indicators representative of their discipline instead of the nursing indicators listed in NOC
• can be reformatted into a nursing goal (outcome statement or expected outcome) when used with its indicators and in conjunction with an expected completion date.

How the taxonomy works

NOC is a five-component classification system that's categorized according to:
• health domain
• outcome class
• outcome labels
• indicators of those outcomes
• measures of the outcomes and indicators.

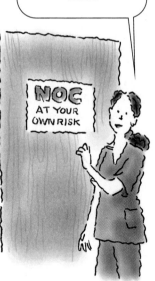

Don't be afraid of NOC. There are several advantages to using the standardized language that NOC offers.

NOC
AT YOUR
OWN RISK

The big breakdown

Seven different domains and 31 classes are identified in NOC. The domains are:
- functional health
- physiologic health
- psychosocial health
- health knowledge and behavior
- perceived health
- family health
- community health.

NOC around the clock

NOC currently includes 330 outcomes, each with its own four-digit taxonomy number, standardized definition, and list of indicators (behavioral criteria by which the more general outcome can be evaluated). To assist in quantifying the behaviors listed, a five-point Likert-type scale is identified for each outcome (see *Get to know Likert scales—Likert or not*, page 100). Users of the system are encouraged, though not mandated, to use the scales provided in order to maintain reliability and validity of outcome measurement. The system also includes a space for the nurse to document an outcome target rating for the patient. (See *Anatomy of a NOC outcome*, page 101.)

Practice your scales

The Likert scales in the NOC system allow nurses (and other clinicians) to evaluate the patient's status from most negative to most positive over time. Examples of scales commonly used to track outcomes include:

Severely compromised 1	Substantially compromised 2	Moderately compromised 3	Mildly compromised 4	Not compromised 5

Never demonstrated 1	Rarely demonstrated 2	Sometimes demonstrated 3	Often demonstrated 4	Consistently demonstrated 5

None 1	Limited 2	Moderate 3	Substantial 4	Extensive 5

Get to know Likert scales—Likert or not

A Likert scale, named after Rensis Likert, is a type of psychometric response scale commonly used in questionnaires. Traditionally, this scale has been used to gauge a participant's level of agreement with a particular statement. For example, a participant might be asked to rate their level of agreement with the statement, "I like ice cream," using a five-point scale that includes "Strongly agree," "Agree," "Neither agree nor disagree," "Disagree," and "Strongly disagree." Each of the categories is assigned a number (for example, "Strongly agree" = 4; "Agree" = 3; "Neither agree nor disagree" = 2, "Disagree" = 1; and "Strongly disagree" = 0) that allows the scale to be scored. Scores for several items are usually combined to provide an overall rating. Likert scales can have more or less than five points; however, five are commonly used. If Likert scales seem familiar to you, you might have encountered them on a course evaluation form.

Ice cream? I strongly agree!

Using NOC to write expected outcomes

Although NOC outcomes aren't the same as expected outcomes, you can use NOC to write outcome statements. Here's how:
• Go to the "NANDA International-NOC Linkages" section of the NOC text and find each of the nursing diagnoses you've selected for your patient. Below each one you'll see the NANDA-International (NANDA-I) definition of the diagnosis and then lists of suggested outcomes and associated outcomes. (See *Speaking the language*, page 102.)
• Choose outcomes from those lists that seem like they might apply to your patient.
• Find each of the potential outcomes in the alphabetical listing in the NOC text, and read the outcome definition and indicators to determine whether the outcome is appropriate for your patient.
• For each appropriate outcome, choose the indicators that apply to your patient.
• Assign baseline ratings for each indicator as well as an overall baseline rating.

Anatomy of a NOC outcome

Becoming familiar with the organization and components of an individual NOC outcome can help you to use NOC to write specific outcome statements for your patients. Below is a sample outcome.

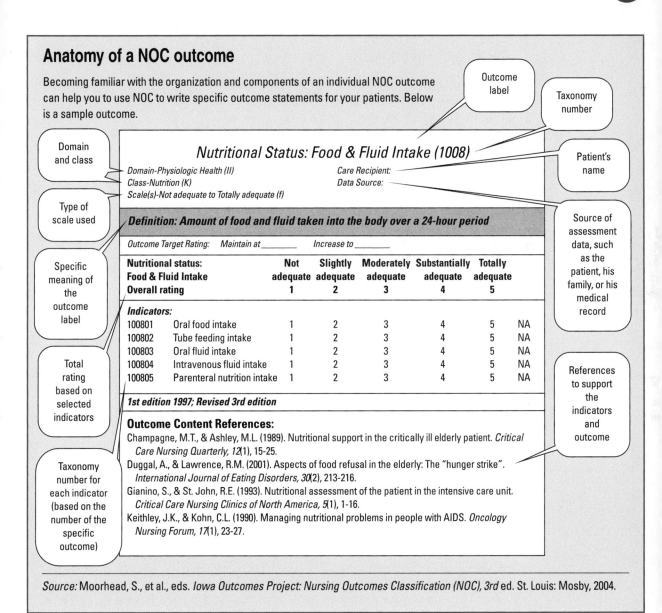

Outcome label

Taxonomy number

Domain and class

Type of scale used

Specific meaning of the outcome label

Total rating based on selected indicators

Taxonomy number for each indicator (based on the number of the specific outcome)

Patient's name

Source of assessment data, such as the patient, his family, or his medical record

References to support the indicators and outcome

Nutritional Status: Food & Fluid Intake (1008)

Domain-Physiologic Health (II)
Class-Nutrition (K)
Scale(s)-Not adequate to Totally adequate (f)

Care Recipient:
Data Source:

Definition: Amount of food and fluid taken into the body over a 24-hour period

Outcome Target Rating: Maintain at _____   Increase to _____

Nutritional status: Food & Fluid Intake Overall rating	Not adequate 1	Slightly adequate 2	Moderately adequate 3	Substantially adequate 4	Totally adequate 5	
Indicators:						
100801 Oral food intake	1	2	3	4	5	NA
100802 Tube feeding intake	1	2	3	4	5	NA
100803 Oral fluid intake	1	2	3	4	5	NA
100804 Intravenous fluid intake	1	2	3	4	5	NA
100805 Parenteral nutrition intake	1	2	3	4	5	NA

1st edition 1997; Revised 3rd edition

Outcome Content References:

Champagne, M.T., & Ashley, M.L. (1989). Nutritional support in the critically ill elderly patient. *Critical Care Nursing Quarterly, 12*(1), 15-25.

Duggal, A., & Lawrence, R.M. (2001). Aspects of food refusal in the elderly: The "hunger strike". *International Journal of Eating Disorders, 30*(2), 213-216.

Gianino, S., & St. John, R.E. (1993). Nutritional assessment of the patient in the intensive care unit. *Critical Care Nursing Clinics of North America, 5*(1), 1-16.

Keithley, J.K., & Kohn, C.L. (1990). Managing nutritional problems in people with AIDS. *Oncology Nursing Forum, 17*(1), 23-27.

Source: Moorhead, S., et al., eds. *Iowa Outcomes Project: Nursing Outcomes Classification (NOC), 3rd* ed. St. Louis: Mosby, 2004.

Speaking the language

Once you start working with the Nursing Outcomes Classification (NOC), you'll quickly realize that the NOC domains are different from the domains listed in NANDA International (NANDA-I) taxonomy. As you'll see later on, both of these domains also differ from the domains in the Nursing Interventions Classification (NIC). The reason for this is that each language is trying to codify a different aspect of nursing care. To successfully incorporate each of these taxonomies into your care plans, be prepared to look at NANDA-I's *Nursing Diagnoses: Definitions & Classification* and the University of Iowa's *Nursing Outcomes Classification (NOC)* and *Nursing Interventions Classification (NIC)* books together. The NOC and NIC books each provide charts to help tie NANDA-I diagnoses into their languages.

Improving for the greater good

In 2000, representatives from NANDA-I, NIC, and NOC created the NNN Alliance, a virtual organization aimed at fostering a working relationship among the three organizations. One goal of this alliance has been to develop a more universal language that can be used not only for these taxonomies but also for other nursing languages.

• Allocate an overall target rating for the patient and a time frame for achieving the goal based on the patient's assessment data, current condition, and personal goals.
(See *NOC outcomes.*)

Developing nursing interventions

Once you've developed expected outcomes for a patient, it's time to start planning specific interventions to achieve them. As with patient outcomes, nursing interventions must be:
• realistic
• measurable
• achievable within the time frame specified in the patient outcome.

Under construction

NOC outcomes

Like all expected outcomes, the outcomes you develop based on the Nursing Outcomes Classification (NOC) should contain the following elements: behavior, measure, criteria, and time frame. However, the form these elements take is modified by the structure of the language of NOC. The examples shown here illustrate two ways in which you might record a NOC expected outcome in your care plan. The actual format you use is determined by your school or facility.

NOC format

This format records the outcome statement in the chart form given in the NOC text.

> Circle the patient's baseline ratings for the indicators that you select here.

> Fill in the patient's target goal rating here. Note that this goal can be either a maintenance goal or an improvement goal.

> Circle the patient's overall baseline rating here.

Nutritional Status: Food & Fluid Intake (1008)

Domain-Physiologic Health (II)
Class-Nutrition (K)
Scale(s)-Not adequate to Totally adequate (f)

Care Recipient: *Susan Wong*
Data Source: *Patient, chart*

Definition: Amount of food and fluid taken into the body over a 24-hour period

Outcome Target Rating: Maintain at _____ Increase to _4_____ *within 1 days*

Nutritional status: Food & Fluid Intake Overall rating	Not adequate 1	Slightly adequate 2	Moderately adequate (3)	Substantially adequate 4	Totally adequate

Indicators:						
100801	Oral food intake	1	2	(3)	4	5	NA
100802	Tube feeding intake	1	2	3	4	5	(NA)
100803	Oral fluid intake	1	2	(3)	4	5	NA
100804	Intravenous fluid intake	1	2	3	4	5	(NA)
100805	Parenteral nutrition intake	1	2	3	4	5	(NA)

1st edition 1997; Revised 3rd edition

Outcome Content References:

Champagne, M.T., & Ashley, M.L. (1989). Nutritional support in the critically ill elderly patient. *Critical Care Nursing Quarterly, 12*(1), 15-25.

Duggal, A., & Lawrence, R.M. (2001). Aspects of food refusal in the elderly: The "hunger strike". *International Journal of Eating Disorders, 30*(2), 213-216.

Gianino, S., & St. John, R.E. (1993). Nutritional assessment of the patient in the intensive care unit. *Critical Care Nursing Clinics of North America, 5*(1), 1-16.

Keithley, J.K., & Kohn, C.L. (1990). Managing nutritional problems in people with AIDS. *Oncology Nursing Forum, 17*(1), 23-27.

Joan Cunningham, RN
3/14/01

> Circle the patient's overall baseline rating here.

> Circle "NA" for any indicators that you haven't chosen for your patient.

> If a copy of the outcome is included in the medical record, sign the outcome and include the date of the assessment.

(continued)

NOC outcomes (continued)

NOC format

This example condenses the information from NOC into a simpler format that is commonly used in schools.

Code or label	Definition and indicators	Measure	Time frame
1008	Nutritional Status: Food & Fluid Intake		
	The amount of food and fluid taken into the		
	body over a 24-hour period		
100801	Oral food intake	at a level of 4 (substantially adequate)	within 1 days
100803	Oral fluid intake	at a level of 4 (substantially adequate)	within 1 days

Remember that you shouldn't change the NOC outcome label and definition; however, you can add new indicators or modify existing ones to make them more specific to your patient. For example, you could redefine the measurement of indicator 100801 of the *Nutritional Status: Food and Fluid Intake* NOC outcome (Oral food intake) to make it more specific (for instance, by defining 1 = No intake, 2 = 25% of food available per meal, 3 = 50% of food available per meal, 4 = 75% of food available per meal, and 5 = 100% of food available per meal).

Types of interventions

Interventions are grouped into two general categories:
- independent
- collaborative (or interdependent).

Independent interventions

An independent intervention is one that falls within the scope of nursing practice. It doesn't require a practitioner's direction or supervision, so you can initiate the action on your own.

You're on your own, kid

Many of the interventions you'll incorporate into the care plan are independent nursing interventions. They address aspects of care that you can do to promote change and facilitate wellness. These interventions cover such topics as:
- performing activities of daily living

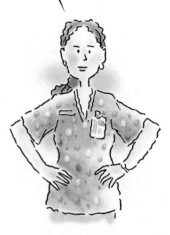

Independent interventions don't require any direction or supervision from a practitioner.

- promoting safety and comfort
- patient teaching.

Independent interventions involve working directly with a patient, such as teaching him how to perform his own insulin injections. However, they also include the indirect activities you pursue to help him reach his goal, such as gathering resource materials about diabetes and insulin self-injection.

Collaborative interventions

A collaborative intervention is one that's based on instructions (oral or written) provided by a practitioner or one that you'll do in consultation with another member of the health care team, such as a dietitian, social worker, or physical therapist. Collaborative interventions fall outside the realm of nursing practice, meaning that you can't initiate them on your own.

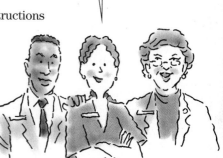

Collaborative interventions are ones that you perform based on the instructions from another member of the health care team.

Hey, let's work together

Examples of collaborative interventions include:
- administering prescribed medications or fluids
- obtaining specimens for laboratory analysis
- inserting catheters.

(See *Comparing independent and collaborative nursing interventions*, page 106.)

Writing nursing interventions

All nursing interventions are based on the goals stated in the patient outcomes and are intended to alter the etiology, defining characteristics, or risk factors for a specific nursing diagnosis. The number of interventions can vary for each outcome. What's most important is that the care plan is comprehensive enough to ensure that the patient can meet the outcomes. You'll usually list several interventions covering various aspects of care, all aimed at correcting the problem identified in the nursing diagnosis.

Each intervention you "prescribe" must be written so that a caregiver (you or another nurse) has a clear picture of what to do to promote a positive change in the patient. As a student, your care plans are generally completed for your instructor, not for the agency or facility where you gain your clinical experience. (See *Tips for writing effective interventions*, page 107.)

Comparing independent and collaborative nursing interventions

Differentiating independent nursing interventions from collaborative interventions can be difficult. Some interventions can be classified as either independent or collaborative, depending on the wording used for the intervention and the nurse's understanding of her scope of practice. One way to differentiate is to consider whether the action is nurse prescribed or practitioner prescribed.

This chart demonstrates a chain of related independent and collaborative nursing actions related to a practitioner order for bed rest.

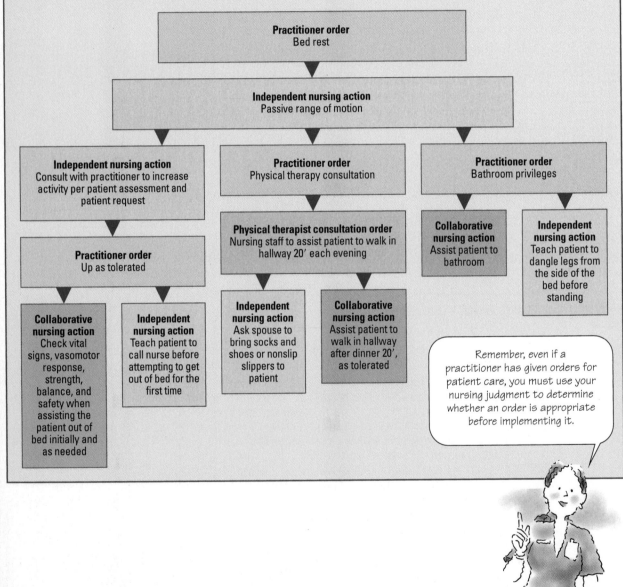

Teacher knows best

Tips for writing effective interventions

To write interventions clearly and correctly, follow these guidelines:
• Keep your interventions simple and to the point, and make sure they're aimed at helping your patient achieve the desired outcome.
• Clearly state the necessary action. Note how and when to perform the intervention, and include special instructions if necessary. For example, "Promote comfort" doesn't tell you what specific action to take, but "Administer ordered analgesic 30 minutes before dressing change" specifies exactly what to do and when to do it.
• Make sure your interventions fit the patient. Consider the patient's age, condition, developmental level, environment, and values. For instance, if the patient is a vegetarian, don't write an intervention that requires him to eat lean meat to gain extra pounds for healing.
• Keep the patient's safety in mind. Consider his physical and mental limitations. For

instance, before teaching a patient how to self-administer medication, make sure he's physically able to do it and that he can remember and follow the regimen.
• Follow your facility's rules. For example, if your facility allows only nurses to administer medications, don't write an intervention calling for the patient to administer hemorrhoidal suppositories as needed.
• Consider other health care activities. Adjust your interventions when other activities interfere with them. For example, you might want your patient to get plenty of rest on a day when he has several diagnostic tests scheduled.
• Use available resources. If your patient needs to learn about his cardiac problem, use your facility's education department, literature from the American Heart Association, and local support groups. Write your intervention to reflect the use of these resources.

> Unlike outcomes, which are patient focused, interventions focus on the actions that you, the nurse, will take.

Identify the activity

Keep in mind that all interventions are actions that *you* (not the patient) will do. Therefore, they should always begin with an action verb, for example:
• <u>Offer</u> fluids every 4 hours.
• <u>Monitor</u> temperature, blood pressure, and pulse.
• <u>Assess</u> pedal pulses.
• <u>Discuss</u> with patient how to perform regular self-breast exams.

Make it specific

Include as many qualifiers as needed to know:
• how, when, and where to do the activity
• how frequently it needs to be done
• special equipment needed
• additional instructions.

Watch the time

Remember that all of the interventions developed for a particular patient outcome must be achievable within the same time frame. This doesn't mean, however, that a particular intervention can't be used again to meet a new progressive outcome related to the original diagnosis.

Keep in mind

When planning interventions, give some thought to:
• likelihood of success, taking into account the timing, interventions by other team members, amount of time required, and cost factors
• resources available to you and your patient
• your ability to perform the intervention
• scientific rationale behind the actions
• the patient's ability and willingness to comply
• prior interventions that you or your patient have successfully used
• interventions from standardized care plans, nursing textbooks, or nursing journals. (See *Plan to succeed.*)

Nursing Interventions Classification

The Nursing Interventions Classification (NIC) is a systematized classification of research-based nursing interventions. NIC interventions cover such areas as illness prevention, illness treatment, and health promotion. Most are designed for individual patients, but some are geared toward families and communities. Covering a broad range of nursing care, NIC may be used in any practice setting and any specialty across the entire health care continuum—from intensive care to primary care, home care, and hospice. Like NOC, NIC is designed so that even nonnurse health care providers can use the interventions in their treatment of patients. The most difficult aspect of using NIC for nurses new to the language is that instead of listing the specific actions the nurse will take, NIC uses labels that group several actions (called *activities*) together.

Class act

NIC consists of 514 interventions (both physiologic and psychosocial labels) that are grouped into 30 classes and 7 domains. The 7 domains are unique to NIC and don't correlate directly with the NANDA-I or NOC domains. They are:
• Physiological: Basic—supports physical functioning
• Physiological: Complex—supports homeostatic regulation

Teacher knows best

Plan to succeed

Always consider your intervention options carefully, and then weigh their potential for success. Determine if you can obtain the necessary equipment and resources. If not, take steps to get what you need or change the intervention accordingly. Also, observe the patient's willingness and functional ability to participate in the various interventions, and be prepared to postpone or modify them if necessary. For example, don't plan extensive verbal teaching with a patient who has significant hearing loss.

- Behavioral—supports social function and lifestyle changes
- Safety—supports protection against harm
- Family—supports the family unit
- Health system—supports use of the health care system
- Community—supports health of the community.

Each intervention in the classification includes a taxonomic code, a label name, a definition, and a list of activities to carry out the intervention. Nurses can select specific activities based on patient need and circumstances. (See *Anatomy of a NIC intervention*, page 110.)

Using NIC to write interventions

Just as you may be asked to use NOC to create your expected outcome statements, you may be asked to choose interventions from a standardized interventions classification, such as NIC. You can find the information in the *Nursing Interventions Classification* book in two ways. First, you can look in the alphabetical listing for the intervention you're interested in. If you find the list daunting or you've looked up what you believe to be key words or concepts for an intervention and haven't found what you wanted, you can search for interventions using NANDA-I nursing diagnoses. *Nursing Interventions Classification* includes charts that list NANDA-I nursing diagnoses alphabetically, with the diagnosis definition and suggested and optional nursing interventions for each diagnosis.

Anatomy of a NIC intervention

Becoming familiar with the organization and components of an individual Nursing Interventions Classification (NIC) intervention can help you to use NIC to write nursing interventions specific to your patients. Below is a sample intervention and its corresponding activities.

Intervention label

Taxonomic code

Definition of label

Feeding   1050

Definition: Providing nutritional intake for patient who is unable to feed self

Activities

Identify prescribed diet

Set food tray and table attractively

Create a pleasant environment during mealtime (e.g., put bedpans, urinals, and suctioning equipment out of sight)

Provide for adequate pain relief before meals, as appropriate

Provide for oral hygiene before meals

Identify presence of swallowing reflex, if necessary

Sit down while feeding to convey pleasure and relaxation

Offer opportunity to smell foods to stimulate appetite

Ask patient reference for order of eating

Fix foods as patient prefers

Maintain patient in an upright position, with head and neck flexed slightly forward during feeding

Place food in the unaffected side of the mouth, as appropriate

Follow feedings with water, if needed

Protect patient's clothing with a bib, as appropriate

Ask the patient to indicate when finished, as appropriate

Record intake, if appropriate

Avoid disguising drugs in food

Provide a drinking straw, as needed or desired

Provide finger foods, as appropriate

Provide foods at most appetizing temperature

Avoid distracting patient during swallowing

Feed unhurriedly/slowly

Postpone feeding, if patient is fatigued

Encourage parents/family to feed patient

Specific activities (suggested activities)

References to support the activities

Background Readings

Evans-Stoner, N.J. (1999). Feeding. In G.M. Bulecheck & J.C. McCloskey (Eds.), Nursing interventions: Effective nursing treatments (3rd ed.) (pp. 31-46). Philadelphia: W.B. Saunders.

Styker, R. (1977). Rehabilitative aspects of acute and chronic nursing care. Philadelphia: W.B. Saunders.

Source: Dochterman, J., and Bulechek, C. *Nursing Interventions Classification (NIC),* 4th ed. St. Louis: Mosby, 2004.

Under construction

Getting the knack of NIC

To better understand NIC, consider this example: You're caring for an elderly man who has Alzheimer's disease. The patient needs assistance with feeding but has no difficulty swallowing.

Using NIC

To determine interventions for this patient using NIC, take a step-by-step approach:
• Determine that the Nursing Outcomes Classification (NOC) entry *Nutritional Status: Food & Fluid Intake* is appropriate for your patient and use this NOC outcome to set outcome goals.
• Look up the corresponding NANDA International diagnosis, *Self-care deficit: Feeding*, in the *Nursing Interventions Classification* book.
• Read through each of the suggested NIC classes that might apply to your patient and choose activities that most closely represent the actions you would need to take, based on your knowledge and research. For example:
   – Environmental management
   – Feeding
   – Nutrition management
   – Oral health maintenance
   – Positioning
   – Self-care assistance: Feeding.
Note: "Bottle feeding" isn't relevant for your patient because he's an adult and "Swallowing therapy" isn't relevant to your patient because he isn't having difficulty swallowing.
• Modify or add to the listed activities as needed. For example:
   – Of the 24 activities, you eliminate seven as not being applicable to your patient.
   – You modify "Protect patient's clothing with a bib, as appropriate" to read "Protect patient's clothing with a cloth napkin" because you know the patient's spouse has brought napkins and this activity conserves the patient's self-esteem.
   – You modify "Record intake, if appropriate" to read "Record fluid intake on I&O sheet; record percentage of food eaten for each meal as 25%, 50%, 75%, or 100%."
   – You add interventions to "Weigh patient weekly," "Monitor trends in weight loss and gain," "Monitor albumin, total protein, and hemoglobin levels and hematocrit as ordered," and "Consult dietitian if patient doesn't respond to interventions by target date."

Personalization

Remember that NIC includes a definition for each class of interventions that shouldn't be changed. However, NIC is designed to be dynamic and flexible, allowing nurses to modify the activities to reflect the unique needs of the patient and his family. Interventions from more than one class may be needed to help the patient achieve his expected outcomes. Nurses can also add activities as appropriate for the patient's particular situation. (See *Getting the knack of NIC.*)

Using evidence-based practice

Evidence-based practice can be defined as the systematic and judicious use of the current best evidence to make decisions about patient care. When applied to nursing, the term *evidence-based practice* is used to describe the care that nurses provide based on research and identified standards.

Shifting sands

Because of the vast amount of available clinical research and accessibility to research findings, there has been a steady shift away from traditional, intuitive-oriented nursing toward evidence-based nursing. Nurses are following the growing trend among all health care fields of using well-designed and executed scientific studies to guide their clinical decision-making and clinical care.

Putting evidence into practice

For your student care plans, your instructor may require you to write rationales for the interventions you've planned or completed. In some cases, students are also required to provide a complete reference list by intervention, or a bibliography.

When planning care, you should use evidence-based research and your critical thinking skills to ascertain why certain actions or practices are being done. Asking pertinent questions can help you determine whether you're taking the right course of action and whether the interventions you've chosen will improve your patient's outcome.

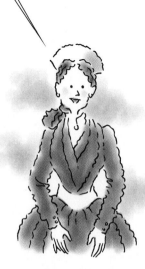

Although tradition has its time and place, evidence-based practice ensures that nurses keep up with the times by using clinically sound best practices.

Don't be afraid to ask

Questions to ask yourself as you plan interventions include:
• Who determined the basis for this treatment?
• What's the rationale for this decision?
• What are the clinical ramifications of this practice?
• Is this the only way of doing this procedure?
• Could this treatment be done better, more efficiently, or more cost-effectively?
• Is this the highest achievable outcome for my patient?

Evaluating sources of information

Truly evaluating the reliability and validity of the findings of a research study requires knowledge of statistics and research principles. However, keeping the following basic principles in mind can help you to identify valid sources of information that can be used to support evidence-based care—and avoid those that don't:

• Check medical resources for guidelines or standards of clinical practice related to your patient's medical diagnosis or the procedures or treatments he may be undergoing.

• Use resources written within the last 3 to 5 years, depending on your faculty's preference.

• Use reputable, well-known journals and textbooks.

• Be wary of research that utilizes small sample sizes because the conclusions from this research may be too narrow to generalize to a larger population.

On the case

Case study background

You're caring for Johanna Keller, a patient with Parkinson's disease. After a recent medication adjustment, the patient's symptoms include mild, bilateral upper extremity tremors that improve with use of the arms and slowed ability to initiate and sustain gross motor movements (such as rising from a bed or chair and walking). The patient is highly motivated to remain as active as possible for as long as possible. Based on her assessment data, you establish the following nursing diagnosis: *Impaired physical mobility related to decreased dopamine neurotransmitter availability (Parkinson's disease) as evidenced by upper extremity tremors and decreased ability to initiate and sustain gross motor movements.*

Critical thinking exercise

1. Based on the definition in the NOC text, you determine that NOC outcome 0208 Mobility (shown on page 114) is appropriate for your patient. Use this NOC outcome to document an outcome statement for this patient.

Mobility (0208)

Domain-Functional Health (I)
Class-Mobility (C)
Scale(s)-Not adequate to Not compromised (a)

Care Recipient:
Data Source:

Definition: Ability to move purposefully in own environment independently with or without assistive device.

Outcome Target Rating: Maintain at _____   Increase to _____

Mobility Overall Rating	Severely compromised 1	Substantially compromised 2	Moderately compromised 3	Mildly compromised 4	Not compromised 5	
Indicators:						
020801 Balance	1	2	3	4	5	NA
020809 Coordination	1	2	3	4	5	NA
020810 Gait	1	2	3	4	5	NA
020803 Muscle movement	1	2	3	4	5	NA
020804 Joint movement	1	2	3	4	5	NA
020802 Body positioning performance	1	2	3	4	5	NA
020805 Transfer performance	1	2	3	4	5	NA
020811 Running	1	2	3	4	5	NA
020812 Jumping	1	2	3	4	5	NA
020813 Crawling	1	2	3	4	5	NA
020806 Walking	1	2	3	4	5	NA
020814 Moves with ease	1	2	3	4	5	NA

1st edition 1997; Revised 3rd edition (formerly Mobility Level)

Outcome Content References:

Gresham, G.E., Duncan, P.W., Stason, W.B., et al. (1995). *Post-stroke Rehabilitation. Clinical practice guideline*, No. 16 (AHCPR Publication No. 95-0062). Rockville, MD: U.S. Department of Health and Human Services. Public Health Services, Agency for Health Care Policy and Research.

Maas, M.L., & Specht, J.P. (2001). Impaired physical mobility. In M. Maas, K. Buckwalter, M. Hardy, T. Tripp-Reimer, M. Titler, & J. Specht (Eds.), *Nursing care of older adults: Diagnoses, outcomes & interventions* (pp. 337-365). St. Louis: Mosby.

McCloskey Dochterman, J., and Bulechek, C. *Nursing Interventions Classification (NIC)*, 4th ed. St Louis: Mosby, 2004.

Podsiadlo, D. & Richardson, S. (1991). The timed "Up & Go": A test of basic functional mobility for frail elderly persons. *Journal of American Geriatrics Society, 39*(2), 142-148.

Rukenstein, L.Z., Wieland, D., & Bernakei, R. (Eds.). (1995). *Geriatric assessment technology: The state of the art*. New York: Springer.

Source: Moorhead, S., et al., eds. *Iowa Outcomes Project: Nursing Outcomes Classification (NOC)*, 3rd ed. St. Louis: Mosby, 2004.

2.   Now review NIC intervention 0226, Exercise Therapy: Muscle Control (shown on page 115). Select at least five nursing activities from this NIC intervention that would be appropriate for this patient.

1.   _____

2.   _____

3.   _____

4.   _____

5.   _____

Exercise Therapy: Muscle Control   0226

Definition: Use of specific activity or exercise protocols to enhance or restore controlled body movement

Activities

Determine patient's readiness to engage in activity or exercise protocol

Collaborate with physical, occupational, and recreational therapists in developing and executing exercise program, as appropriate

Consult physical therapy to determine optimal position for patient during exercise and number of repetitions for each movement pattern

Evaluate sensory functions (e.g., vision, hearing, and proprioception)

Explain rationale for type of exercise and protocol to patient/family

Provide patient privacy for exercising, if desired

Adjust lightning, room temperature, and noise level to enhance patient's ability to concentrate on the exercise activity

Sequence daily care activities to enhance effects of specific exercise therapy

Initiate pain control measures before beginning exercise/activity

Dress patient in nonrestrictive clothing

Assist patient to maintain trunk and/or proximal joint stability during motor activity

Apply splints to achieve stability of proximal joints involved with fine motor skills, as prescribed

Reevalutate need for assistive devices at regular intervals in collaboration with PT, OT, or RT

Assist patient to sitting/standing position for exercise protocol, as appropriate

Reinforce instructions provided to patient about the proper way to perform exercises to minimize injury and maximize effectiveness

Determine accuracy of body image

Reorient patient to body awareness

Reorient patient to movement functions of the body

Coach patient to visually scan affected side of body when performing activities of daily living (ADLs) or exercises, if indicated

Provide step-by-step cues for each motor activity during exercise or ADLs

Instruct patient to "recite" each movement as it is being performed

Use visual aids to facilitate learning how to perform ADLs or exercise movements, as appropriate

Assist patient to develop exercise protocol for strength, endurance, and flexibility

Assist patient to formulate realistic, measurable goals

Use motor activities that require attention to and use of both sides of the body

Incorporate ADLs into exercise protocol, if appropriate

Encourage patient to practice exercises independently, as indicated

Assist patient with/encourage patient to use warm-up and cool-down activities before and after exercise protocol

Use tactile (and/or tapping) stimuli to minimize muscle spasm

Assist patient to prepare and maintain a progress graph/chart to motivate adherence to exercise protocol

Monitor patient's emotional, cardiovascular, and functional responses to exercise protocol

(continued)

Activities:—cont'd

Monitor patient's self-exercise for correct performance

Evaluate patient's progress toward enhancement/restoration of body movement and function

Provide positive reinforcement for patient's efforts in exercise and physical activity

Collaborate with home caregivers regarding exercise protocol and ADLs

Assist patient/caregiver to make prescribed revisions in home exercise plan, as indicated

Background Readings

Donohue, K., Miller, C., & Craig, B. (1988). Chronic alterations in mobility. In P.H. Mitchell, L.C. Hodges, M. Muwaswes, et al. (Eds.), AANN's neuroscience nursing: Phenomena and practice (pp. 319-343), Norwalk, CT: Appleton & Lange.

Glick, O.J. (1992). Interventions related to activity and movement. In G.M. Bulechek & J.C. McCloskey (Eds.), Symposium on Nursing Interventions. Nursing Clinics of North America, 27(2) 541-568.

Hickey, J. (1992). The clinical practice of neurological and neurosurgical nursing (3rd ed.). Philadelphia: J.B. Lippincott.

Hogue, C. (1985). Mobility. In E.G. Schneider et al. (Eds.), The teaching nursing home. New York: Raven Press.

Lewis, C.B. (1989). Improving mobility in older persons. Rockville, MD: Aspen.

Lubkin, I. (1990). Chronic illness: Impact and intervention (2nd ed.). Boston: Jones & Bartlett.

McCloskey Dochterman, J., and Bulechek, C. Nursing Interventions Classification (NIC), 4th ed. St Louis: Mosby, 2004.

McFarland, G.K., & McFarlane, E.A. (1997). Nursing diagnosis and intervention. (3rd ed.). St. Louis: Mosby.

Moorhouse, M., Geissler, A., & Doenges, M. (1987). Critical care plans, guidelines for patient care. Philadelphia: F.A. Davis.

Pender, N.J. (1987). Health promotion nursing practice (2nd ed.). Norwalk, CT: Appleton & Lange.

Sullivan, P., & Markos, P. (1993). Clinical procedures in therapeutic exercise. Norwalk, CT: Appleton & Lange.

Vogt, G., Miller, M., & Esluer, M. (1985). Mosby's manual of neurological care. St. Louis: Mosby.

Source: Dochterman, J., and Bulechek, C. Nursing Interventions Classification (NIC), 4th ed. St. Louis: Mosby, 2004.

Out or in?

Read each statement. On the blank line provided, write "O" if the statement is an outcome or write "I" if it's an intervention.

_____ 1. Assist with ambulation, as needed.

_____ 2. Demonstrate proper use of ambulation with quad cane within 4 days of discharge.

_____ 3. Administer oral analgesics three times per day, as prescribed.

_____ 4. Monitor vital signs every 4 hours until stable.

_____ 5. Offer sips of water and ice chips, as tolerated, followed by soft diet by HD 2 postop.

_____ 6. Maintain acceptable body weight throughout length of stay.

_____ 7. Provide environmental cues (clock, calendar, pictures) to assist with orientation.

_____ 8. Encourage participation in daily self-care.

_____ 9. Avoid straining when having a bowel movement throughout hospitalization.

_____ 10. Verbalize decreased pain as evidenced by lower score on pain-rating scale within 1 week.

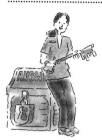

Answer key

Critical thinking exercise

1. The NOC outcome statement for this patient might look like this:

Mobility (0208)

Domain-Functional Health (I)
Class-Mobility (C)
Scale(s)-Not adequate to Not compromised (a)

Care Recipient: *Johanna Keller*
Data Source: *Patient, chart*

Definition: Ability to move purposefully in own environment independently with or without assistive device.

Outcome Target Rating: Maintain at _____ Increase to __4__ *within 3 days*

Mobility Overall Rating	Severely compromised 1	Substantially compromised 2	Moderately compromised 3	Mildly compromised 4	Not compromised 5	
Indicators:						
020801 Balance	1	2	3	4	5	(NA)
020809 Coordination	1	2	3	(4)	5	NA
020810 Gait	1	2	3	(4)	5	NA
020803 Muscle movement	1	2	3	(4)	5	NA
020804 Joint movement	1	2	3	4	5	(NA)
020802 Body positioning performance	1	2	3	4	5	(NA)
020805 Transfer performance	1	2	3	(4)	5	NA
020811 Running	1	2	3	4	5	(NA)
020812 Jumping	1	2	3	4	5	(NA)
020813 Crawling	1	2	3	4	5	(NA)
020806 Walking	1	2	3	(4)	5	NA
020814 Moves with ease	1	2	3	4	5	(NA)

1st edition 1997; Revised 3rd edition (formerly Mobility Level)

Outcome Content References:

Gresham, G.E., Duncan, P.W., Stason, W.B., et al. (1995). *Post-stroke Rehabilitation. Clinical practice guideline*, No. 16 (AHCPR Publication No. 95-0062). Rockville, MD: U.S. Department of Health and Human Services. Public Health Services, Agency for Health Care Policy and Research.

Maas, M.L., & Specht, J.P. (2001). Impaired physical mobility. In M. Maas, K. Buckwalter, M. Hardy, T. Tripp-Reimer, M. Titler, & J. Specht (Eds.), *Nursing care of older adults: Diagnoses, outcomes & interventions* (pp. 337-365). St. Louis: Mosby.

McCloskey Dochterman, J., and Bulechek, C. *Nursing Interventions Classification (NIC)*, 4th ed. St Louis: Mosby, 2004.

Podsiadlo, D. & Richardson, S. (1991). The timed "Up & Go": A test of basic functional mobility for frail elderly persons. *Journal of American Geriatrics Society, 39*(2), 142-148.

Rukenstein, L.Z., Wieland, D., & Bernakei, R. (Eds.). (1995). *Geriatric assessment technology: The state of the art*. New York: Springer.

Source: Moorhead, S., et al., eds. *Iowa Outcomes Project: Nursing Outcomes Classification (NOC)*, 3rd ed. St. Louis: Mosby, 2004.

2.   Examples of nursing activities that would be appropriate for this patient include:
- Determine patient's readiness to engage in activity or exercise protocol
- Collaborate with physical, occupational, and recreational therapists in developing and executing exercise program, as appropriate
- Consult physical therapy to determine optimal position for patient during exercise and number of repetitions for each movement pattern
- Explain rationale for type of exercise and protocol to patient/family
- Sequence daily care activities to enhance effects of specific exercise therapy
- Reevalutate need for assistive devices at regular intervals in collaboration with PT, OT, or RT
- Reorient patient to movement functions of the body
- Assist patient to develop exercise protocol for strength, endurance, and flexibility
- Incorporate ADLs into exercise protocol, if appropriate
- Evaluate patient's progress toward enhancement/restoration of body movement and function

Note that other nursing activities may also be appropriate.

Out or in?

1. Intervention
2. Outcome
3. Intervention
4. Intervention
5. Intervention
6. Outcome
7. Intervention
8. Intervention
9. Outcome
10. Outcome

Implementation

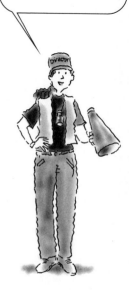

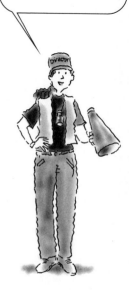

Less talk,
more action.
Implementation is the
time to put your care
plan into action.

Just the facts

In this chapter, you'll learn:

♦ responsibilities associated with implementation of a care plan

♦ strategies for gathering and organizing patient information

♦ methods for integrating care activities

♦ the importance of communicating with the interdisciplinary team

♦ two commonly used documentation methods.

Implementation overview

Once you've written a care plan—including the nursing diagnoses, patient outcomes, and interventions needed to achieve those outcomes—you're ready to put the care plan into action.

Let's get hands-on

Implementation, the fourth step in the nursing process, is the step during which you'll have hands-on involvement with your patient. It encompasses:
• employing planned interventions
• using your critical thinking skills to solve problems and set priorities
• continually reassessing the patient's response to your interventions
• communicating effectively with other members of the health care team
• documenting all of the care you provide.

All in a day's work

To implement a care plan, expect to perform some or all of the following types of interventions:
• routine assessment and monitoring of the patient
• therapeutic interventions, such as administering medications or obtaining ordered specimens
• offering comfort measures
• providing nourishment
• helping with activities of daily living
• supporting respiratory and elimination functions
• providing skin care
• offering emotional support
• providing patient teaching and counseling
• communicating with other interdisciplinary team members.

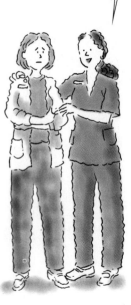

Don't be afraid to ask. If you need help, consult with other nursing staff before you perform an intervention.

Somebody point me in the right direction!

It's normal to feel slightly overwhelmed and even frightened when you begin implementing your nursing care plan, especially if you're a nursing student or are just beginning your nursing career. However, this lack of confidence will dissipate with time and ongoing experience. Remember, the care plan is a road map to helping your patient achieve wellness. It will point you in the direction toward achieving that goal, but it's your responsibility to determine if you need additional information or help from other staff before implementing an intervention.

Levels of responsibility

Your role in preparing and implementing a nursing care plan will vary with your level of nursing experience.

Student body

As a nursing student, your goal is to work from a care plan that you develop based on your assessment of the patient. In reality, you might not have access to your patient or his medical record until shortly before you become responsible for providing his care. In this situation, you need to review the care plan already in place as a blueprint for implementation. As you complete your own patient assessment, you become responsible for modifying the established care plan to reflect any changes and implementing your new interventions. The care plan you later write for your instructor may include diagnoses and interventions you actually had no time to initiate in the confines of your clinical time with the patient. (See *Who's the boss?* and *The nursing shortage*, page 122.)

Who's the boss?

As a nursing student, you're likely to feel like you have too many masters. In the classroom and laboratory settings, you must follow the directions of your instructor. However, clinical rotations can be much more confusing because you'll receive instruction from multiple members of the health care team. Understanding each person's role and practicing some basic skills can help you to work successfully with all team members in this challenging situation.

Clinical instructors

Commonly, clinical instructors are part-time faculty members who are paid by nursing schools to supervise students in a clinical setting. They also commonly work part-time at the various hospitals or agencies where they supervise students. This gives them knowledge of the structure and function of that particular setting and a relationship with the nursing staff, practitioners, managers, and other professionals with whom students might interact.

Clinical instructors are responsible for supervising the direct patient care students provide, using a skill proficiency checklist. For example, every student is required to demonstrate competence in medication administration via each route of administration before being permitted to independently obtain and administer drugs to a patient. Skills practiced in simulation labs may also require demonstration. Instructors question students during the day on all facets of their knowledge, planning, implementation, and documentation of care in order to assess basic understanding of nursing care provision and critical thinking skills.

Clinical site staff

In addition to your clinical instructor, you will also be responsible for frequent and open communication with the patient's primary nurse. Remember, the staff nurse assigned to the patient bears overall responsibility for verifying that all required nursing actions are completed in a safe and timely manner, in accor-

dance with the patient's care plan. The staff member assigned to the patient must know exactly which aspects of care you'll be providing, whether you might need supervision or assistance with a skill (in case the clinical instructor isn't immediately available), and the results of your assessments and actions.

A learning experience

When you're on your clinical rotations, you may feel that you waste a lot of time looking for the staff nurse or your clinical instructor, leaving barely enough time to get your skills checked off and your work done. Use this frustrating situation to practice building some personal skills that will benefit you throughout your nursing practice, such as:
• flexibility—what else can you be looking up, cleaning up, finishing up, writing up, or setting up while you wait?
• assertiveness—who else can answer your question or solve your patient's need, where else can you look for the information you need, how else can you correctly but politely convey the time frame or degree of urgency you're working under?
• coping ability—what else can you do to defuse your anxiety and frustration right now, how else can you think about this experience that will help you learn something useful about how nurses function day to day on the job, when else can you practice communicating honestly with a patient without off-loading your tension or anger onto him?

> Do clinical rotations have your head spinning? Take a minute to remind yourself what each person's role is.

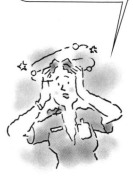

The nursing shortage

One of the many ways the nursing shortage is affecting health care is the increasing shortage of nursing instructors. You may notice that this shortage directly impacts your nursing education and clinical practice.

On campus

On your campus, the instructor shortage may be reflected by the increased use of part-time educators rather than full-time teachers. This change means that you get to know more nurses who have insights to share, but you may also have more trouble accessing an instructor when you have questions or problems with your studies. It may also mean that schools can't expand to try to fill the need for nurses.

In clinicals

In the clinical setting, the shortage of instructors can significantly limit your access to the types of experience you need in order to function comfortably and satisfactorily as a new graduate. The effects of the nursing instructor shortage are complicated by other changes in the health care industry, including the shortening of admission times for acute care, home health care, and rehabilitation patients. Advances in medical technology and knowledge have made minimally invasive surgical and diagnostic techniques with shorter recovery times much more common and increased the number of procedures that can be done in a short procedure unit. Cost containment practices by health insurers have also contributed to a decrease in available time to support and educate patients. Each of these changes means fewer opportunities for new nurses to interact with and care for patients.

Because of this growing crisis, researchers are working with educational institutions and health care institutions to try out new models of clinical education. You may hear about some of the following solutions being used in your school:

• Clinical partnerships—Experienced baccalaureate-level staff registered nurses are trained as clinical adjunct instructors and supervise the clinical assignments and experiences of a small cadre of students. The assigned faculty member supervises two or more adjunct instructors and facilitates the clinical experience.

• Clinical preceptorships—Experienced staff registered nurses with demonstrated teaching ability are partnered one-on-one with a student for a semester and guide them through their clinical objectives while modeling nursing in the real world. The student coordinates her clinical experiences with the preceptor's work schedule. The faculty member coordinates the program, mentors the preceptors, and supervises all aspects of the clinical experience.

• Joint student experiences—Junior and senior level students work together on a unit, with seniors taking turns as team leader. Juniors perform interventions to their skill level and are mentored by senior students. Seniors obtain experience in delegation and management as well as senior level skills. Instructors from each level team up to provide clinical supervision.

• Alternative clinical settings—Students gain their clinical experience in a variety of community health settings that haven't traditionally been used for this purpose, such as public health clinics, prisons, Native American reservations, museums, community service agencies, churches, and senior centers. Even international settings have been used in some schools. A staff person from the agency is trained as a preceptor and assists the student in selecting appropriate projects to meet the clinical course requirements. Faculty members supervise the overall program and meet with each student and site regularly.

• Alternative clinical requirements—Faculty redesign clinical experiences to more closely match real-world nursing experiences. All preclinical preparation is eliminated. Students are required to research drugs just prior to administration; chart reviews and initial care plans are done during the clinical day. Only relevant laboratory and diagnostic tests must be reported, the physical examination is streamlined, and documentation consists primarily of checklists. The goal is to reduce wasted time and effort and focus on productivity, time management skills, and attainment of clinical skills.

Graduate fellowship

As a practicing nurse, you'll initially follow a care plan developed by another nurse, and you may not know much about the patient before you actually meet him and begin providing care. Your game plan remains the same as when you were a student, though—modify the care plan as needed as you develop your own assessment data. As you're given new patients to admit to the unit, you'll have opportunities to develop complete care plans for them.

Regardless of your place in the nursing hierarchy, it's up to you to learn as much as you can about your patient and his current condition before implementing care. You're even responsible for making sure that a practitioner's orders are appropriate for a patient before you implement them.

Getting started

Start your implementation of the care plan by assessing the patient's current situation. Then gather the supplies you'll need to complete the planned interventions.

Assessing the situation

Even if this is your first encounter with this patient, a great deal of information about the patient is available to you from various sources. For example, you can gather plenty of useful information by:
• listening to the report of the departing nurse at the start of your shift
• reading the patient's chart, including information obtained during the initial history and physical examination
• talking with other staff, including your clinical instructor and the patient's primary nurse
• talking with the patient and family members
• directly observing and assessing the patient
• reviewing laboratory and other test results.

Shifting gears

Begin your shift by listening to the previous shift nurse's report about the patient. (See *Bedside shift report—A new model*, page 124.) On a worksheet, write any pertinent information about the patient's vital signs, activities, intake and output, frequency of treatment, and special instructions.

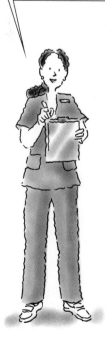

Write it down! The more information you write down, the more data you have to reference later on.

Weighing the evidence

Bedside shift report—A new model

New research highlights the benefits of conducting the shift report at the patient's bedside. In addition to professional nurses, unlicensed assistive personnel can also attend the report. The research documents increases in patient satisfaction with their overall care, oncoming nurses' satisfaction with their information about patients' needs and status, physician satisfaction with the nurses' knowledge about their patients, and management's satisfaction with the decreased amount of overtime required per shift.

Source: Anderson, C., and Mangino, R. "Nurse Shift Report: Who Says You Can't Talk in Front of the Patient?" *Nursing Administration Quarterly* 30(2): 112-22, April-June 2006.

If you work in a setting that has an electronic health record system, you may be able to print a patient-specific report of all orders and test results from the system. Some systems also contain the nursing care plans. (See *Sample electronic shift report.*)

Take note of this

After listening to report, you should review the patient's chart for any new orders that may have been written. Note any changes in the patient's treatment or care regimen on both the care plan and your worksheet. Also review the medication and I.V. fluid administration record, and make notes (on your worksheet) of the times that medications, I.V. fluids, and other I.V. drugs are scheduled. Note the frequency of treatments, vital signs, dressing changes (and type), and blood glucose monitoring. This will help you to organize and integrate your planned independent nursing interventions with the collaborative interventions listed in the care plan.

Making contact

Next, assess the patient. After entering the patient's room, introduce yourself, wash your hands, and then check the patient's identification. Remember to use two patient identifiers, such as his name, birth date, or assigned identification number. Whenever possible, ask the patient to tell you his name instead of calling him by his name. (See *National Patient Safety Goals*, page 128.)

Perform your initial assessment and make notes of your findings; these notes will provide the basis for your initial nurse's note in the patient's medical record. You can also use this opportunity to talk briefly with the patient (and any family members who may

> It's a good idea to highlight medication and I.V. administration times on your worksheet.

Sample electronic shift report

Many electronic health record systems are programmed to send practitioners' medical orders directly to the staff who will be implementing them. For example, new medication orders are sent to the pharmacy-specific section of the record system as well as to the nursing-specific section. Staff members in these departments can print out information they need to know from the records and use it to plan their work. Nurses usually obtain a printout (or electronic shift report) on each of their assigned patients at the start of their shifts. They might also regularly check the computer for new orders throughout their shift.

Although electronic shift reports are valuable, they shouldn't be used in place of verbal shift reports because the data they provide about a patient's current status are limited. For example, electronic reports don't tell you how your patient is doing, what issues are most important for follow-up, or what the last assessment revealed. The electronic shift report printout is a good place to make notes about information obtained during the verbal shift report.

Here's a sample electronic nursing shift report.

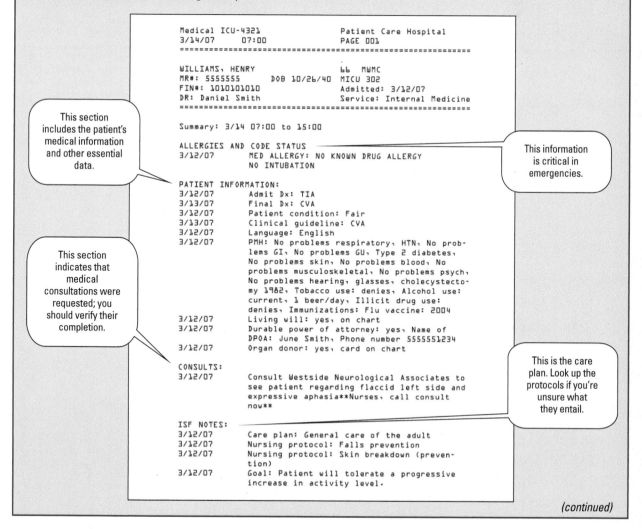

This section includes the patient's medical information and other essential data.

This information is critical in emergencies.

This section indicates that medical consultations were requested; you should verify their completion.

This is the care plan. Look up the protocols if you're unsure what they entail.

```
Medical ICU-4321              Patient Care Hospital
3/14/07      07:00            PAGE 001
==================================================================

WILLIAMS, HENRY                    66  MWMC
MR#: 5555555        DOB 10/26/40  MICU 302
FIN#: 1010101010                  Admitted: 3/12/07
DR: Daniel Smith                  Service: Internal Medicine
==================================================================

Summary: 3/14 07:00 to 15:00

ALLERGIES AND CODE STATUS
3/12/07        MED ALLERGY: NO KNOWN DRUG ALLERGY
               NO INTUBATION

PATIENT INFORMATION:
3/12/07        Admit Dx: TIA
3/13/07        Final Dx: CVA
3/12/07        Patient condition: Fair
3/13/07        Clinical guideline: CVA
3/12/07        Language: English
3/12/07        PMH: No problems respiratory, HTN, No prob-
               lems GI, No problems GU, Type 2 diabetes,
               No problems skin, No problems blood, No
               problems musculoskeletal, No problems psych,
               No problems hearing, glasses, cholecystecto-
               my 1982, Tobacco use: denies, Alcohol use:
               current, 1 beer/day, Illicit drug use:
               denies, Immunizations: Flu vaccine: 2004
3/12/07        Living will: yes, on chart
3/12/07        Durable power of attorney: yes, Name of
               DPOA: June Smith, Phone number 5555551234
3/12/07        Organ donor: yes, card on chart

CONSULTS:
3/12/07        Consult Westside Neurological Associates to
               see patient regarding flaccid left side and
               expressive aphasia**Nurses, call consult
               now**

ISF NOTES:
3/12/07        Care plan: General care of the adult
3/12/07        Nursing protocol: Falls prevention
3/12/07        Nursing protocol: Skin breakdown (preven-
               tion)
3/12/07        Goal: Patient will tolerate a progressive
               increase in activity level.
```

(continued)

Sample electronic shift report *(continued)*

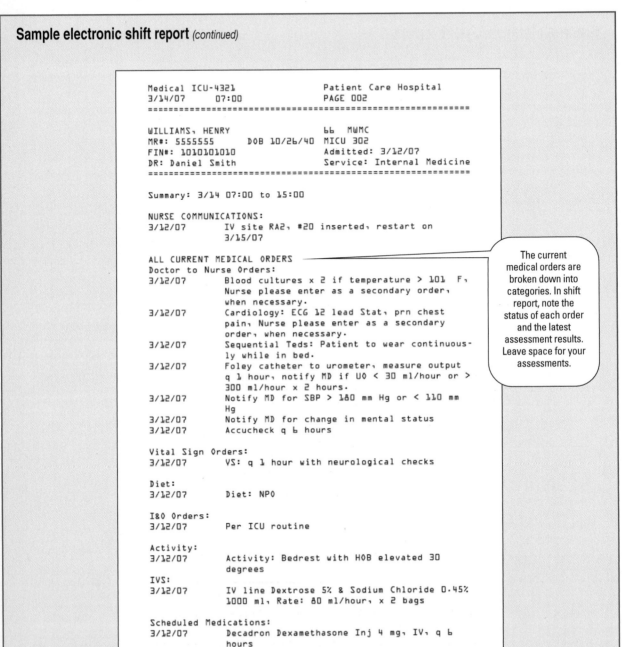

```
Medical ICU-4321            Patient Care Hospital
3/14/07     07:00           PAGE 002
===============================================================

WILLIAMS, HENRY                 66   MWMC
MR#: 5555555       DOB 10/26/40 MICU 302
FIN#: 1010101010                Admitted: 3/12/07
DR: Daniel Smith                Service: Internal Medicine
===============================================================

Summary: 3/14 07:00 to 15:00

NURSE COMMUNICATIONS:
3/12/07        IV site RA2, #20 inserted, restart on
               3/15/07

ALL CURRENT MEDICAL ORDERS
Doctor to Nurse Orders:
3/12/07        Blood cultures x 2 if temperature > 101  F,
               Nurse please enter as a secondary order,
               when necessary.
3/12/07        Cardiology: ECG 12 lead Stat, prn chest
               pain, Nurse please enter as a secondary
               order, when necessary.
3/12/07        Sequential Teds: Patient to wear continuous-
               ly while in bed.
3/12/07        Foley catheter to urometer, measure output
               q 1 hour, notify MD if UO < 30 ml/hour or >
               300 ml/hour x 2 hours.
3/12/07        Notify MD for SBP > 180 mm Hg or < 110 mm
               Hg
3/12/07        Notify MD for change in mental status
3/12/07        Accucheck q 6 hours

Vital Sign Orders:
3/12/07        VS: q 1 hour with neurological checks

Diet:
3/12/07        Diet: NPO

I&O Orders:
3/12/07        Per ICU routine

Activity:
3/12/07        Activity: Bedrest with HOB elevated 30
               degrees
IVS:
3/12/07        IV line Dextrose 5% & Sodium Chloride 0.45%
               1000 ml, Rate: 80 ml/hour, x 2 bags

Scheduled Medications:
3/12/07        Decadron Dexamethasone Inj 4 mg, IV, q 6
               hours
                    09        15
```

The current medical orders are broken down into categories. In shift report, note the status of each order and the latest assessment results. Leave space for your assessments.

Sample electronic shift report *(continued)*

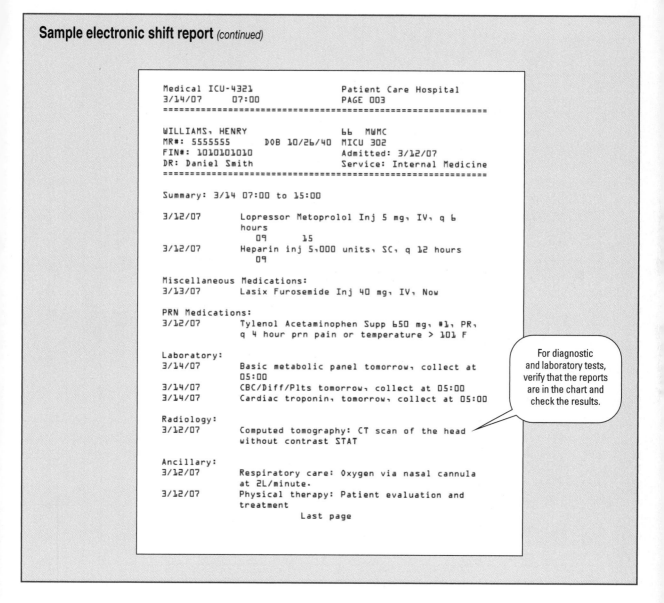

```
Medical ICU-4321              Patient Care Hospital
3/14/07      07:00            PAGE 003
================================================================

WILLIAMS, HENRY                  66  MWMC
MR#: 5555555      DOB 10/26/40   MICU 302
FIN#: 1010101010                 Admitted: 3/12/07
DR: Daniel Smith                 Service: Internal Medicine
================================================================

Summary: 3/14 07:00 to 15:00

3/12/07         Lopressor Metoprolol Inj 5 mg, IV, q 6
                hours
                    09       15
3/12/07         Heparin inj 5,000 units, SC, q 12 hours
                    09

Miscellaneous Medications:
3/13/07         Lasix Furosemide Inj 40 mg, IV, Now

PRN Medications:
3/12/07         Tylenol Acetaminophen Supp 650 mg, #1, PR,
                q 4 hour prn pain or temperature > 101 F

Laboratory:
3/14/07         Basic metabolic panel tomorrow, collect at
                05:00
3/14/07         CBC/Diff/Plts tomorrow, collect at 05:00
3/14/07         Cardiac troponin, tomorrow, collect at 05:00

Radiology:
3/12/07         Computed tomography: CT scan of the head
                without contrast STAT

Ancillary:
3/12/07         Respiratory care: Oxygen via nasal cannula
                at 2L/minute.
3/12/07         Physical therapy: Patient evaluation and
                treatment
                        Last page
```

> For diagnostic and laboratory tests, verify that the reports are in the chart and check the results.

be present if the patient gives permission) and gather additional information about the patient's:

• perception of his current illness and his overall health and well-being

• ability to perform the interventions to meet the outcomes specified in the care plan

• available resources and support system.

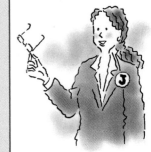

Weighing the evidence

National Patient Safety Goals

Since July 2002, The Joint Commission has annually published National Patient Safety Goals that they require an organization to meet before it can be accredited. These standards, or goals, are developed based on safety statistics, research, and input from numerous health care professionals and consumers. The validity of the goals is so well recognized that many institutions follow them even if they aren't seeking accreditation.

A few of the important safety goals you might need to implement in your clinical settings are:
• using at least two forms of patient identification before initiating any care, service, or treatment
• engaging in a pause before the start of any invasive procedure (called a *time out*) in which all staff actively confirm that the right patient is present, the right procedure is scheduled, and that the right site for the procedure has been marked
• eliminating all nonstandardized abbreviations and symbols in medical communications
• complying with your facility's standardized system for giving and receiving shift report, which includes the opportunity for questions and answers
• labeling all medications and medication containers
• labeling all laboratory specimens in the presence of the patient
• reconciling the patient's medication list with the admission list before admission and then communicating his current medication list on discharge to all health care providers involved in his aftercare and, in writing, to the patient himself
• assessing each patient's risk of falls and implementing a program to reduce this risk
• assessing each patient's risk of health care–associated pressure ulcers and implementing a program to reduce this risk
• assessing each patient's inherent risks, such as a patient with an emotional or a behavioral disorder being regularly assessed for suicide or a home care patient on oxygen therapy being assessed for the risk of fire.

Source: The Joint Commission. "National Patient Safety Goals." Available at *www.jointcommission.org/PatientSafety/NationalPatientSafetyGoals/*.

Student report

If you're a student, provide a brief verbal report of your findings to the patient's assigned nurse and your clinical instructor, alerting them immediately to any abnormal findings. Ask them to clarify anything you're unsure about or ask your clinical instructor to check on the patient to verify your findings. (See *Nurses as resources.*)

Teacher knows best

Nurses as resources

Experienced nurses can be an invaluable resource. They've amassed a wealth of information through practical experience in providing bedside care. They can teach you organizational skills and strategies for thinking through situations that you may encounter in the clinical setting. Tapping into their knowledge can help you to fine-tune your assessment and care techniques in your quest to become a registered nurse.

Gathering supplies

After you've performed your initial assessment, you'll gather and assemble the appropriate equipment and supplies for other interventions you'll need to perform. Once you've properly prepared yourself and the necessary supplies, it's time to implement your care.

Providing care

Now you're ready to begin tackling specific interventions. Being prepared and developing a system that integrates various activities can save you time and benefit your patient by reducing interruptions to his rest.

Basic implementation steps

Although the specific care activities that you'll perform will depend on the patient's condition, some general practices apply to all patients. The timing of meals, therapies, tests, and procedures the patient is scheduled to receive will determine which of the other interventions specified in the care plan you'll initiate next.

Meet Mr. Med

When your patient is due to receive a medication, locate and prepare the medications under the supervision of your nursing instructor or the patient's primary nurse. (See *Safe drug administration guidelines*, page 130.) Follow a tried-and-true set of safeguards known as the "five rights" to help you avoid the most basic

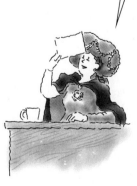

I see medication administration in your future. Make sure that you have the right drug, dose, patient, time, and route.

Teacher knows best

Safe drug administration guidelines

When administering a drug, be sure to adhere to best practices to avoid potential problems and manage those that do occur. You can help prevent drug errors by following these guidelines as well as facility policy.

Drug orders
• Don't rely on the pharmacy computer system to detect all unsafe orders. Before you give a drug, understand the correct dosage, indications, and adverse effects.
• Be aware of the drugs your patient takes regularly, and question any deviation from his regular routine. As with any drug, take your time and read the label carefully.
• Before you give drugs that are ordered in units, such as insulin and heparin, always check the prescriber's written order against the provided dose. Never abbreviate the word "units."
• To prevent an acetaminophen overdose from combined analgesics, note the amount of acetaminophen in each drug. Beware of substitutions by the pharmacy because the amount of acetaminophen may vary.

Drug preparation and administration
• Always check the expiration date before administering a drug.
• If a familiar drug has an unfamiliar appearance, find out why. If the pharmacist cites a manufacturing change, ask him to double-check whether he has received verification from the manufacturer. Document the appearance discrepancy, your actions, and the pharmacist's response in the patient record.
• Use two patient identifiers, such as the patient's name and assigned identification number, to identify the patient before administering any drug or treatment. Teach the patient to offer his identification bracelet for inspection when anyone arrives with drugs and to insist on having it replaced if it's removed.
• Ask the patient to verify his allergy history before administering an antibiotic.
• Ask the patient about his use of alternative therapies, including herbs, and record your findings in his medical record. Monitor the patient carefully and report unusual events. Ask the patient to keep a diary of all therapies he uses and to take the diary for review each time he visits a health care professional.

Avoiding common problems
Calculation errors
• Writing the milligrams per kilogram (mg/kg) or milligrams per meter squared (mg/m^2) dose and the calculated dose provides a safeguard against calculation errors. Whenever a prescriber provides the calculation, double-check it and document that the dose was verified.
• Don't assume that liquid drugs are less likely to cause harm than other forms. Pediatric and geriatric patients commonly receive liquid drugs and may be especially sensitive to the effects of an inaccurate dose. If a unit-dose form isn't available, calculate carefully and double-check your math and the drug label.
• Read the label on every drug you prepare and never administer any drug that isn't labeled.

Air bubbles in pump tubing
• To clear bubbles from I.V. tubing, never increase the pump's flow rate to flush the line. Instead, remove the tubing from the pump, disconnect it from the patient, and use the flow-control clamp to establish gravity flow.
• When the bubbles have been removed, return the tubing to the pump, restart the infusion, and recheck the flow rate.

Incorrect administration route
• When a patient has multiple I.V. lines, label the distal end of each line.
• Never use a parenteral syringe to prepare oral liquid drugs (this increases the chance for error because the syringe tip fits easily into I.V. ports). To safely give an oral drug through a feeding tube, use a dose prepared by the pharmacy and a syringe with the appropriate tip.

and common medication errors. Each time you administer a medication, confirm that you have the:

- right drug
- right dose
- right patient
- right time
- right route.

Room service

At meal times, raise the head of the bed so that the patient can sit upright. Adjust his tray, and assess his need for fresh water. Ask about any special requests, such as the desire for juice or other food items. Place the call bell within the patient's reach, and instruct him to call you with any additional needs or concerns.

Before you leave

Each time you prepare to exit the patient's room, look over your care plan and worksheet. Identify the interventions you've completed, and make note of any changes to the care plan that need to be made. Also note any changes in the patient's status, his response to treatment and care, and his refusal of care, treatments, or regimens (all of which require nursing note entries in the patient's medical record).

Status report

Report any abnormal findings, patient or family concerns, changes in the patient's condition, or uncertainty or concern about findings to your clinical instructor and the patient's primary care nurse. Also report your completion of ordered treatments and regimens.

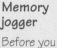

Memory jogger

Before you administer a drug, remember your nursing responsibilities for this intervention. To remember the sequence of the actions you must take, think "Until Clear, Ask Many Times":

Understand the drug and how it works.

Clarify the drug order as needed.

Administer the drug.

Monitor the patient for therapeutic response to the drug and for adverse effects.

Teach the patient about the drug as needed.

Integrating activities

Although you could approach each intervention separately when providing care, systematically checking off each intervention in the care plan, this approach isn't the most practical use of your time and energy. A more effective approach is to try completing as many interventions as possible during each visit to the patient's room. Coordinating and integrating your nursing care between or with activities of daily living, medication administration, vital signs assessments, treatments, and other collaborative and interdependent care has several benefits:

- It saves time.
- It enhances your coordination skills.
- It allows you to provide efficient and timely care.

When taking an integrated approach, remember to review your care plan and notes carefully because you'll be attempting to complete several interventions during a single visit.

Implementation example

Because the care that you provide is specific to each patient, a sample scenario might help you to better understand ways in which you can successfully integrate routine activities to implement efficient patient care. Suppose you're working the morning shift (7 a.m. to 3 p.m.) in a hospital and you're assigned a patient with a neuromuscular impairment. After report, you review the care plan, which included the nursing diagnoses:
• *Self-care deficit (bathing and hygiene) related to neuromuscular impairment and generalized debility as evidenced by inability to wash body and obtain bath supplies*
• *Risk for impaired skin integrity related to decreased mobility and poor nutritional intake*
Your nursing care plan for this patient might look like the one shown in *Understanding implementation: Sample care plan.*

Based on the care plan, interventions for this patient may include:
• taking vital signs
• administering ordered morning medications
• assisting with morning hygiene (such as bathing, oral care, toileting, and grooming)
• assessing skin, diet, fluid intake, musculoskeletal strength, and mobility
• changing the bed linens
• positioning the patient
• providing a nutritious breakfast.

You'll also need to incorporate other assessments, such as assessment of cardiopulmonary status, bowel elimination, and pain, into your care to gain a full picture of the patient's status.

Making the most of your time

Remember, to provide the most effective care possible, you may need to integrate several interventions. Here are some ways in which you can integrate the caregiving tasks that you need to perform:
• If the patient's ability allows, ask him to wash his face while you're setting up supplies for his bed bath. Observe the patient's reaction to this request and the action taken in response to assess the patient's interest in self-care, ability to understand and follow instructions, functional use and range of motion (ROM) of upper extremities, and signs of discomfort.

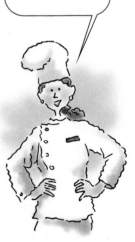

Mealtimes are another good opportunity to assess your patient's status and his needs.

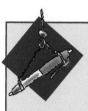

Under construction

Understanding implementation: Sample care plan

This sample care plan was developed for a patient who has problems with bathing and hygiene and who's at risk for skin breakdown because of his chronic illness and current hospitalization.

Date	Nursing diagnosis	Patient outcomes	Interventions	Outcome evaluation (initials and date)
5/8/01	Self-care deficit (bathing and hygiene) related to neuromuscular impairment and generalized debility as evidenced by inability to wash body and obtain bath supplies	• The patient will wash his face, arms, frontal trunk, and perineal area on morning shift by discharge. • The family will demonstrate safe and effective assistance with patient's bath and hygiene on morning shift by discharge.	• Assess the patient's functional level every shift, and document findings. • Assist with or perform bathing daily while promoting patient independence in bathing the parts of his body within his reach and his maximal functional ability. • Change linens daily and as needed. • Assess the family's knowledge of proper bath and linen change procedures, safety measures, and rationale for personal hygiene in order to meet the patient's bathing and hygiene needs on discharge. • Instruct the family as needed on safe techniques for providing bathing and hygiene needs. • Observe family members demonstrate safe and effective assistance with the patient's personal care. • Assess the family's need for home care assistance to provide the patient's bathing and hygiene needs for safety or respite issues. • Refer the patient to social services, as needed, for assistance in obtaining home support services.	

REVIEW DATES		
Date	**Signature**	**Initials**
5/8/01	Jackie Miller, RN	JM

(continued)

Understanding implementation: Sample care plan (continued)

Date	Nursing diagnosis	Patient outcomes	Interventions	Outcome evaluation (initials and date)
5/8/01	Risk for impaired skin integrity related to decreased mobility and poor nutritional intake	• The patient will remain free from skin breakdown during the hospital stay. • The patient will maintain adequate food and fluid intake during the hospital stay. • The family will demonstrate proper use and understanding of home measures to prevent skin breakdown by discharge.	• Assess skin integrity every shift and as needed. • Assess dietary and fluid preferences on admission. • Assess dietary intake and fluid intake and output every shift. • Assess the family's knowledge of principles and practices of skin care and their need for specialized equipment to promote good care at home. • Keep skin and linens clean and dry, and keep linens wrinkle-free. • Turn and reposition the patient every 2 hours and as needed. • Apply lotion to dry skin areas after bathing, at bedtime, and as desired by the patient. • Provide foods and fluids of choice that are nutritionally appropriate for the patient's diet and medical regimen. • Promote patient intake of at least 1 L of noncaffeinated liquids per day. • Teach the family as needed about skin care and observation techniques, position change requirements, and nutritional and fluid needs to prevent skin breakdown. • Observe the family demonstrate and verbalize understanding of all instructions given. • Refer the patient to a dietitian for protein and calorie evaluation, as needed. • Refer the patient to social services for assistance in obtaining special equipment in the home, as needed.	

REVIEW DATES

Date	Signature	Initials
5/8/01	Jackie Miller, RN	JM

• While the patient washes himself, ask about pain or discomfort with movement, level of fatigue, usual activity level before this hospitalization, the availability of people to assist him at home, and any preferences for skin care.
• While helping the patient shave, assess endurance and fine motor skills and ROM of the hands and arms.
• When applying lotion to the patient's hands, assess bilateral grip strength, radial pulses, capillary refill, and gross sensory disturbances.
• While washing the patient's lower extremities, assess strength and ROM of legs and feet, endurance, skin integrity, distal pulses, capillary refill, toenails, and gross sensory disturbances.
• While helping the patient wash his perineal area, discuss bowel and bladder status or problems and observe skin integrity of the abdomen and groin.
• While assisting with oral hygiene, assess the teeth, gums, tongue, and oral mucosa and encourage the patient to drink sufficient amounts of water. Teach the importance of adequate fluid intake to maintain healthy skin and bowel and bladder function.

Working with the interdisciplinary team

Nurses aren't the only health care professionals involved in patient care. As you implement care, you'll need to collaborate with an interdisciplinary team to meet the diverse needs of your patients.

Share and share alike

The focus of an interdisciplinary team is on the patient and patient outcomes. Each team member shares responsibility for achieving these outcomes. To provide more effective and comprehensive care, you need to understand each team member's role. (See *Meet the interdisciplinary team*, page 136.)

Passing notes is permitted

When you're reviewing the patient's chart, be sure to read the progress notes written by other members of the health care team. Those notes will provide you with important information about your patient.

Remember, patient care is a team sport.

Meet the interdisciplinary team

Members of the interdisciplinary health care team—and their roles—include:
• physician, physician's assistant, nurse practitioner, and consultant specialty physicians—who assess, monitor, and provide treatment guidelines for the patient's medical conditions
• primary nurse, advanced practice or clinical nurse specialist, and nurse-manager—who assess, monitor, teach, and intervene to help the patient meet his expected outcomes by discharge
• registered dietitian—who assesses and monitors nutritional needs
• social worker—who provides support and counseling to patients and their families and helps with financial difficulties
• occupational therapist—who assists the patient in performing activities of daily living, participating in recreation, and working to the highest functional level
• physical therapist—who assists the patient to improve or restore physical functioning and prevent deconditioning
• respiratory therapist—who monitors and provides airway management
• pastoral care specialist—who provides religious and spiritual support to patients and their families
• pharmacist—who reviews, prepares, and dispenses the patient's medications; provides information and guidance in the preparation and administration of medications; and provides patient education (in an outpatient setting)
• discharge planner—who coordinates access to ongoing services after discharge, such as transfer to another facility, arrangement for medical equipment in the home, or referral for home health services.

Hospice or palliative care
In a hospice or palliative care setting, the interdisciplinary team would also include:
• volunteer—who provides emotional and diversional support and respite to the patient and family
• bereavement counselor—who supports and counsels the family for 1 year after the death of the patient.

Important reminder
And don't forget the most important members of the team: the patient and his family. No interventions can occur and no goals can be met unless the patient permits the care and is committed to the outcome.

If you have questions about the patient's condition or treatment, contact the appropriate team members for more information. For example, a pharmacist can tell you how to space medications to eliminate drug or food interactions, whereas a physical therapist can provide you with written instructions on the patient's prescribed exercises.

Play well with others

You'll also need to coordinate care with other team members. For example, medicating your postoperative patient before respiratory exercises helps the patient cough and deep breathe more effectively with the respiratory therapist. When working with other team members, remember to use good communication skills. Above all, treat all team members with respect, and they'll respect you in turn!

Documenting interventions

Documentation is an important component of implementation. As previously mentioned, you should take notes after each intervention you perform, including the nature of the intervention, the time you performed it, and the patient's response as well as interventions you performed based on the patient's response and the reasons you performed them. Each intervention should also be documented in the patient's medical record. You should record interventions whenever you:
- give routine care
- give emergency care
- observe changes in the patient's condition
- administer medications
- perform procedures or interventions.

Tailor-fit to house style

Where do you document your interventions? That depends on your facility's policy. You can document them on graphic records, on a patient care flow sheet that integrates all nurses' notes for a 1-day period, on integrated or separate nurses' progress notes, and on other specialized documentation forms (such as the medication administration record). Your facility's policies also dictate the style and format of the documentation.

Focused documentation

Your documentation should be patient-centered and outcome-oriented. Stating the patient's response to your nursing interventions help to make your documentation patient-centered. Linking your interventions and responses to the nursing diagnoses and goal statements makes it outcome-oriented as well.

Documentation formats

Various types of nursing note formats are used in the clinical setting. They may be done by hand or in a computerized charting system. Two of the most commonly used formats for documenting interventions are discussed here.

PIE system

The problem-intervention-evaluation (PIE) system organizes information according to patient problems and was devised to simplify the documentation process. This system requires you to keep a daily patient assessment flow sheet and to write structured progress notes.

Piecing PIE together

Each piece of PIE has it's own purpose:
• The problem category is used to identify the nursing diagnosis requiring the interventions.
• The intervention category describes the actions you took and any assessment data related to the interventions.
• The evaluation section describes the results of your interventions and any additional information regarding attaining your outcomes. (See *Using PIE documentation.*)

SOAP format

SOAP is an acronym for subjective data, objective data, assessment, and planning. The SOAP system, which is used in problem-oriented medical record charting, allows all health care team members to record their findings using narrative progress notes. This system allows readers to readily distinguish between the subjective and objective data so the correct plan of care can be chosen, and you can show that your interventions addressed the patient's documented needs. It also specifies the follow-up care that's planned.

Using PIE documentation

For the nursing diagnosis *Self-care deficit: Bathing and hygiene,* you would document your care using the PIE format in this way:

P—Self-care deficit: Bathing and hygiene

I—Assisted pt. with bath; he was able to wash his own hands and upper chest slowly without discomfort.
Pt. unable to lift arms above chest; muscle strength grade 3/6 upper and lower extremities. Remains on
practitioner-ordered bed rest. Changed linens and repositioned pt. onto left side after applying oil-based
lotion to skin.

E—Continues to require major assistance with personal care. Plan to assess the family's ability to meet
the pt.'s bathing and hygiene needs when they visit in the afternoon.

For the nursing diagnosis *Risk for impaired skin integrity,* you would document your care using the PIE format in this way:

P—Risk for impaired skin integrity

I—Pt. assessment revealed warm, dry skin that's papery on the lower legs with some flaking. Sacral area is
reddened from lying supine, but color clears when the patient is repositioned onto left side. No other areas
of redness or any other defects present. Radial, dorsalis pedis, and posterior tibial pulses +2 and equal
bilaterally; all nail beds show brisk capillary refill. Applied lotion after bath. Pt. ate 50% of breakfast;
states "I don't get too hungry anymore. I like a hot breakfast but I don't care for bacon or sausage, just
eggs or oatmeal". Instructed pt. that dietitian can visit and help him choose meals he likes as well as find
ways to keep up his protein and calories so his skin remains healthy. Pt. agreeable but requests visit in
the afternoons, when his wife is here. Also taught pt. importance of drinking 4 to 6 cups of noncaffeinated
fluids per day for skin, bowel, and bladder health and applying lotion to dry extremities, particularly the
lower legs, at least twice daily.

E—Pt. verbalized understanding of all instructions but prefers to have wife hear information as well; pt.
states "she keeps track of everything now." Pt. offers to ask her to rub lotion on his legs and arms during
her afternoon visits. Referral made to dietitian.

The dirt on SOAP

To use the SOAP format, document the following information for each problem:

• Subjective data: Information the patient or family members tell you, such as the chief complaint

• Objective data: Factual, measurable data you gather during assessment, such as vital signs and laboratory test results

• Assessment data: Conclusions based on the collected subjective and objective data and formulated as patient problems and nursing diagnoses; these conclusions are dynamic, changing as more or different data become known

• Plan: Your strategy for relieving the patient's problem, including both short- and long-term measures.

(See *Using SOAP notes.*)

Using SOAP notes

For the patient problem *Self-care deficit: Bathing and hygiene,* you would document your care using the SOAP format in this way:

> S—"I can't get to my bath supplies because my strength is gone. I can't even move myself."
>
> O—Pt. unable to lift arms above chest. Washed own hands and upper chest slowly. Muscle strength grade 3/6 upper and lower extremities. Pt. remains on practitioner-ordered bed rest.
>
> A—Self-care deficit: Bathing and hygiene
>
> P—Continue to provide for pt.'s bathing and hygiene needs. Assess and instruct family regarding alternate methods for meeting bathing and hygiene needs.

For the patient problem *Risk for impaired skin integrity,* you would document your care using the SOAP format in this way:

> S—"I'm feeling some pressure and pain in my lower back."
>
> O—Papery dry skin on the lower legs with some flaking; sacral area reddened from lying supine.
>
> A—Risk for impaired skin integrity
>
> P—Continue to change position frequently. Apply lotion to dry areas.

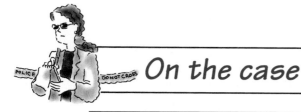

On the case

Case study background

For your first clinical rotation on a medical-surgical unit, you're assigned to care for two patients. Your first patient is Shirley Trotter, a 75 year old who was admitted yesterday with pneumonia and severe shortness of breath. Your second patient is Carl Conrad, a 46 year old admitted 3 days ago for an abdominal cholecystectomy.

Critical thinking exercise

To help prepare for your clinical experience, place these steps in proper sequence by numbering them from 1 to 9:

_____ A. Assess Shirley Trotter.

_____ B. Document your care and the patients' responses to your interventions.

_____ C. Receive the shift report from your patients' previous nurse.

_____ D. Greet your patients, introduce yourself to them, and verify their identities per protocol.

_____ E. Check in with your instructor and prepare the patients' morning medications, gathering any other supplies needed.

_____ F. Receive your patient assignment, research the medical diagnoses and existing care plans, and establish preliminary priorities of care.

_____ G. Assess Carl Conrad.

_____ H. Review medication and I.V. fluid administration records.

_____ I. Complete as many interventions as possible during each visit to each patient's room.

_____ J. Administer your patients' morning medications.

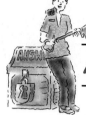

Answer key

Critical thinking exercise
1. F, 2. C, 3. H, 4. D, 5. A, 6. G, 7. E, 8. J, 9. I, 10. B

Evaluation

6

Just the facts

In this chapter, you'll learn:

♦ the importance of continually reassessing the patient's condition during all phases of care

♦ criteria for evaluating care

♦ the process for evaluating whether a care plan must be revised and the way in which revisions should be implemented.

A look at evaluation

Although designated as the fifth phase of the nursing process, evaluation is really an ongoing practice that occurs with every patient encounter. It encompasses:
• reassessing the patient
• comparing your findings with the outcome criteria established in the care plan
• determining the extent of the patient's progress, or outcome achievement (whether an outcome goal was met, partially met, or not met)
• writing evaluation statements
• revising the care plan, including nursing diagnoses, outcomes, and interventions, as needed
• documenting your evaluation.

The value of evaluation

Each evaluation you make depends primarily on your ability to form an opinion or judgment about the data you collect. As a nurse, you'll use your evaluation findings to:
• determine if the original assessment findings still apply to the patient's condition
• uncover complications

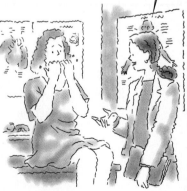

Don't be nervous about being evaluated. Evaluation is an ongoing and critical part of patient care.

- assess and analyze trends or patterns in the patient's response to all aspects of his care, including medications, changes in diet or activity, procedures, unusual incidents or problems, and teaching
- determine how closely your care conforms to established standards
- assess the results of care provided by other health care team members
- identify opportunities to improve the quality of care.

Reassessing a patient

Reassessment is a necessary part of evaluation. After all, how else can you determine whether your patient's condition is improving, your interventions are working, or your patient is making sufficient progress toward achieving his outcome goals?

The patient and the process

It's important to note that reassessment includes not only periodically rechecking your patient's status throughout his care but also reexamining all phases of the nursing process in relation to the patient. This involves reviewing all the nursing diagnoses, patient outcomes, and specific interventions written into the care plan. (See *Evaluation throughout the nursing process.*)

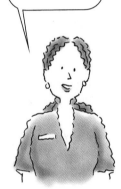

Reassessment is a necessary part of evaluation.

Comparing patient data

In order to evaluate care, you must first compare your patient's prior assessment data to your follow-up assessment data to see whether his condition has changed. This comparison allows you to make inferences about the patient's condition and to alter the care plan accordingly.

Data déjà vu

When comparing data, remember to review all the patient's findings, including:
- his baseline level of functioning at the time of admission
- his most recent assessment findings
- any other pertinent data collected within the past 24 hours.

Your comparison should include a careful review of the patient's functional level, vital signs, and general overall status.

Evaluation throughout the nursing process

Assessment, or more correctly *reassessment*, takes place at all phases of the nursing process. Examples of the types of questions you can ask as you move through the stages of the nursing process are shown below. Remember that any change in the patient's condition that's outside of the expected findings requires you to notify the practitioner.

Nursing process step		Questions
Assessment		Have the patient's vital signs changed? What's the patient's current pain scale rating?
Nursing diagnosis		Is this diagnosis still relevant? Do the current signs and symptoms point to any new diagnoses?
Planning		Are the outcomes still realistic in the time allotted? Do the interventions still match the patient's expected outcomes?
Implementation		Did I observe a response when I implemented the interventions? Was the patient comfortable with the interventions?
Evaluation		How do the reassessment findings compare with the original findings? Can I document the nursing diagnostic goal as met?

Begging the question

Next, you should compare the patient's current condition with his condition prior to the initiation of care to determine his response to your interventions (independent and collaborative). Ask yourself these two key questions:

How is my patient responding to care?

What's his current condition (is he stable, improving, or worsening)?

Your answers to these questions will help guide your decisions about follow-up care. (For an example of how to evaluate patient data, see *Is my patient improving?*, page 146.)

Report, record, react

The follow-up care you'll perform will be determined by the results of your reassessment evaluation. If the patient's condition is stable or improved, your next step is documentation of your findings. If, however, you feel the patient's condition is remaining stat-

Is my patient improving?

You've been working with an elderly, bedbound, terminally ill patient. One of the major nursing considerations for this patient is his comfort level, which includes keeping him free from painful skin breakdown.

Initial assessment
The patient's initial assessment showed:
• very dry, flaking skin on the lower legs and feet
• buildup of dead skin on the soles
• deep-red heels that are continuously tender
• present and equal dorsalis pedis and posterior tibial pulses bilaterally
• absence of edema
• sluggish capillary refill.

A nursing diagnosis of *Impaired skin integrity related to immobility, decreased nutrition, and skin effects of aging* was identified on the patient's care plan, which also included the following expected outcomes:
• The skin on the patient's lower extremities will be pink, dry, and intact by discharge.
• The patient's skin will be free from additional areas of impaired skin integrity throughout hospitalization.

Your assessment
Your assessment on day 3 of admission reveals:
• soft skin on the lower legs and feet
• slight flaking of the skin on the ankles and feet
• decrease of 50% in residual dead skin buildup
• deep-red heels that are tender to touch
• unchanged pulses, edema, and capillary refill.

Comparing assessments
When you compare the new data you collected to the initial patient data, you determine that the patient's condition is improving and your plan is to continue to implement the nursing interventions identified on the care plan and to continue to monitor the patient. If your assessment had revealed that the patient's condition was unstable or worsening, in addition to continuing with established interventions you may also add new interventions, such as consulting the practitioner and wound care specialist for additional treatments or requesting an order for a specialty bed.

ic or deteriorating, be prepared to suggest the next appropriate actions and give your rationales for them. Then proceed with further interventions as appropriate. Keep in mind that you'll need to document your findings and the care plan revisions. As a student nurse, you'll also need report your assessment data to the primary nurse and your instructor.

Teacher knows best

Keeping track of interventions

One suggestion for keeping track of the interventions you perform is to check off the interventions after you perform them, and then write down data that suggest the patient is making progress toward achieving the goal. Also remember to evaluate and document in your notes how the patient tolerates the interventions you perform and any unexpected effects related to the intervention.

Evaluating interventions and goals

At some point, you'll need to conduct a systematic review of all your interventions to gauge your patient's progress toward achieving the expected outcomes. When you do this, you'll ask yourself many additional questions, such as:
• Do the reassessment findings show that the interventions are working?
• Are some interventions no longer necessary?
• Have any or all of the patient's short-term goals been met? Have long-term goals been met?

Complete or communicate

As a student, you might not be able to perform all of the interventions included in a patient's care plan. However, you're responsible for communicating to your instructor and the patient's primary care nurse which interventions you did and did not complete. (See *Keeping track of interventions.*) This communication ensures that the patient's primary care nurse knows what interventions still need to be completed so that the patient receives all of the planned nursing interventions.

Achieving expected outcomes

On evaluation, you may determine, based on the patient's response to treatment and care, that the patient has met his short-term goals. For example, you may have successfully employed all of the interventions needed to return your patient's assessment findings to within normal limits. Hence, your evaluation would lead you to assume that the expected outcome has been met.

To help clarify this concept, consider a practical real-life example, such as buying a new pair of shoes. (See *The blue shoe blues,* page 148.)

The blue shoe blues

Here's a practical example of how to evaluate whether expected outcomes have been met: Imagine that you've been invited to a party to celebrate your completion of nursing school. You have a beautiful, new blue dress at home that you've been saving for just such an occasion. However, you assess your shoe wardrobe and are sad to discover that you have no blue shoes to match the dress. Your nursing diagnosis (note that this one isn't NANDA International approved) is *Shoe deficit, blue*. Your short-term goal is to buy a new pair of blue shoes right away that are comfortable and reasonably priced. You remember that the shoe store down the street is having a sale, and you drive there to search for shoes that are just the right color, size, and price. You make your purchase—a new pair of blue suede shoes—and drive home happy.

So, from a nursing perspective, how would you evaluate what you've just done? In this example, the best approach is to compare the diagnosis to the goal to determine what you've accomplished. The flowchart below takes you through this process step by step.

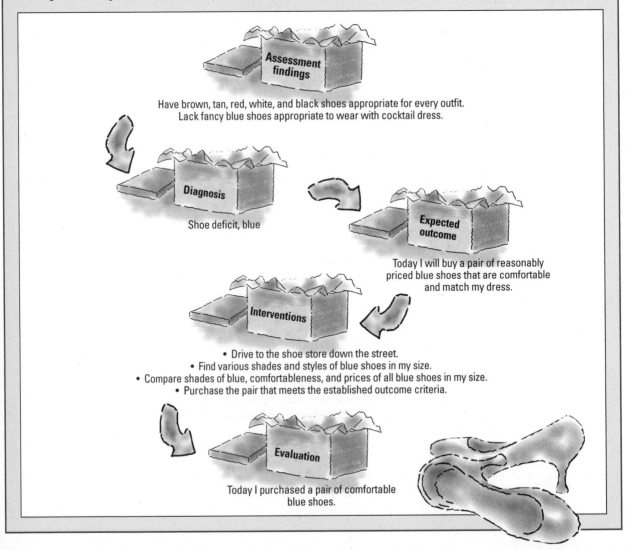

Assessment findings

Have brown, tan, red, white, and black shoes appropriate for every outfit.
Lack fancy blue shoes appropriate to wear with cocktail dress.

Diagnosis

Shoe deficit, blue

Expected outcome

Today I will buy a pair of reasonably priced blue shoes that are comfortable and match my dress.

Interventions

• Drive to the shoe store down the street.
• Find various shades and styles of blue shoes in my size.
• Compare shades of blue, comfortableness, and prices of all blue shoes in my size.
• Purchase the pair that meets the established outcome criteria.

Evaluation

Today I purchased a pair of comfortable blue shoes.

When expected outcomes aren't met

Achieving expected outcomes indicates progress in your patient's care. However, suppose that you perform all of the interventions in the care plan and your patient's condition doesn't improve or, worse yet, his condition has deteriorated. These findings indicate that the expected outcomes haven't been achieved. So, what do you do? At this point, you must reassess the situation.

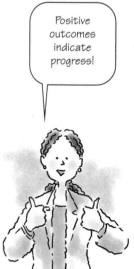

Positive outcomes indicate progress!

A case of intolerable interventions?

You're caring for a 78-year-old patient with a nursing diagnosis of *Self-care deficit: Toileting related to weakness as evidenced by muscle strength 4/6 in lower extremities, a prior order for bed rest, and loss of muscle mass due to aging.* This patient's expected outcome is that he will ambulate to the bathroom with assistance the third day after admission. You begin performing the following interventions, as mentioned in the care plan:
• Assess the patient's functional level and strength before getting him out of bed.
• Dangle the patient's feet at the side of the bed before assisting him to a standing position.
• Assist the patient out of bed to the bathroom when needed.
• Instruct the patient to call for assistance with toileting before an urgent need, and explain planned interventions to achieve the expected outcome.

As soon as you begin assisting the patient to sit on the side of the bed to dangle his legs, you hear him state that he feels dizzy. You immediately help him to lie back down in bed and take these vital signs: blood pressure 80/58 mm Hg, pulse 110 beats/minute, and oxygen saturation per pulse oximetry 97% on room air. You check these measurements and find that the patient's morning vital signs were: blood pressure 110/64 mm Hg, pulse 88 beats/minute, and oxygen saturation per pulse oximetry 97% on room air. These vital sign changes and the patient's complaint of dizziness lead you to conclude that the patient's condition has changed. Given the circumstances, he's unable to carry out the intervention and, therefore, can't meet his expected outcome.

Reassess the patient's condition to determine whether the intervention you performed (assisting the patient to dangle his legs before standing) caused the response (dizziness, tachycardia, and hypotension) or whether the response is a sign or symptom of a worsening condition or a complication. Ask yourself the following questions:
• Is this response a continuation or exacerbation of an existing problem or condition?

• Is this response due to something that has changed in the patient's condition?
• Is this a new problem that needs to be addressed by a revision of the care plan?

Subtle signs

During evaluation, always pay attention to even slight changes in assessment findings. Sometimes, a mild physiologic adaptation, such as a response to a position change, can mimic a subtle change in condition. Because of a relative lack of clinical experience, student nurses commonly have difficulty making such distinctions, which can affect the care plans they create for patients. Remember, when you're in doubt, you and your patient will benefit most if you ask for help from another nurse or from your instructor.

The power of reassessment

When evaluation reveals changes in a patient's condition or expected outcomes that haven't been achieved by the nursing interventions set out in the care plan or when your interventions create an unexpected patient response that leads to new symptoms or a worsening of the patient's condition, you must reassess not only the patient but also your expectations for the patient (expected outcome). In some cases, the care plan will need to be revised to reflect a different patient outcome and a new set of interventions.

Documenting changes

Remember to write a nurse's note (electronic or handwritten) that describes the patient's changed condition. Use the format preferred by your facility for this note. Also document any calls that you make to the practitioner to inform him of changes in the patient's condition, including the time the call was made.

Writing evaluation statements

Part of the evaluation process involves writing a statement that describes whether the patient has achieved the expected outcome (short- or long-term goal) as it was written into the care plan.

Revisiting goals

As you may recall, short-term goals are those that can be accomplished during the patient's hospital stay (usually within 1 week or less), whereas long-term goals are those that can be accomplished over an extended time (usually more than 1 week).

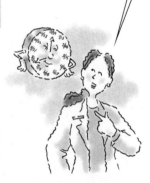

Short-term goals are those that can be accomplished during the patient's hospital stay, usually within a week.

May I *opine?*

Your evaluation statement should indicate whether the expected outcome was achieved. However, your documentation just prior to the evaluation statement should list the evidence supporting this conclusion. This evidence is the information you obtained in your reassessment and evaluation. These conclusions can state that an outcome has been fully met, partially met, or not met.

Write right

In your actual charting, your evaluation should contain three types of information:
• results of your reassessment
• results of your comparison of the reassessment data with the patient's baseline data or normal findings
• evaluation statement that specifies the patient's status toward achieving his expected outcomes.

Evaluating short-term goals

Your evaluation of a short-term goal should occur within the time-frame established in the patient outcome statement. You should determine the patient's progress toward achieving the goal within the time-frame and revise the care plan if needed. Keep in mind that your patient may have more than one short-term goal for each nursing diagnosis.

Let's walk through it together

For example, if a patient outcome states that "The patient will ambulate in the hallway two times with minimal assistance on the evening shift on 6/22/07," you must evaluate the patient's progress toward accomplishing that goal by the end of your shift on that day. If the patient fails to achieve the goal by the end of your shift, you must document this in your nursing notes in the form of an evaluation statement, such as "Patient was unable to tolerate second attempt at ambulating in hallway with assistance; expected outcome not met." Of course, your reassessment data supporting this evaluation would be documented in the chart according to the format used in the facility.

Evaluating long-term goals

Your patient's long-term goal may be the desired end-result of nursing care or, in some cases, a goal that extends beyond the usual time-frame of his hospital stay. Such conditions as stroke, myocardial infarction, traumatic brain injury, neurologic or spinal

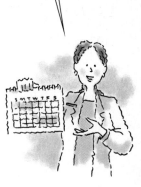

Long-term goals take more time to accomplish— sometimes weeks or months.

injury, hip fracture, and Alzheimer's disease commonly require long-term goals that extend over a continuum of care. Typically, patients with these conditions are discharged from the hospital to a long-term care facility or home health agency for continued nursing treatment and care.

Taking the long road home

For example, the patient with a nursing diagnosis of *Self-care deficit: Toileting related to weakness as evidenced by muscle strength 4/6 in lower extremities, a prior order for bed rest, and loss of muscle mass due to aging* may have the following expected outcome: "Ambulate to bathroom with minimal assistance within 1 month after discharge to nursing rehabilitation center."

Such a goal establishes a clear timeline for evaluating the outcome (within 1 month) and sets the criteria (with assistance, after discharge from the hospital or transfer to the rehabilitation center).

Evaluating the care plan

In addition to periodically evaluating the patient's status and progress toward achieving outcomes, you'll also need to evaluate the care plan in its entirety. This means going through each section of the plan to determine whether the patient's problems have been resolved, outcomes have been achieved, and interventions are still appropriate and current.

> Reevaluating the care plan is just as important as reevaluating the patient.

Reviewing the plan

Your reassessment of the care plan will yield much information about what you and the patient have accomplished and what care still needs to be done. Ask yourself the following questions, taking each section in turn.

Look at the nursing diagnoses

- Does the patient still have the same problems (nursing diagnoses)? If so, has the focus of any of the problems changed in a way that would warrant rewriting the diagnosis?
- Were the diagnoses confirmed or ruled out?
- Does the patient have any new needs? If so, should any additional diagnoses be added to the care plan?
- Are all of the diagnoses prioritized?

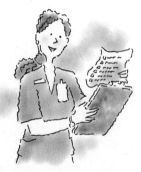

Check patient outcomes

- Has the patient achieved the short- and long-term outcomes for each nursing diagnosis?
- Is each goal still valid and achievable within its given time frame?
- Should the care plan include any additional criteria for achieving the outcomes?
- Does the patient agree with the stated outcomes?
- If the patient didn't achieve the outcomes, do you know why?

Review the interventions

- Do the interventions address the patient's specific needs?
- Are they achievable within the designated time frames?
- Are they clearly written so that other team members can follow them?
- Should any interventions be discontinued or rewritten?

Evaluating the plan

Once you've reviewed the care plan, you can provide a written evaluation (on the care plan itself or in your progress notes) of each care plan section. Be sure to base your evaluation on information gathered from all sources, including your own observations and findings, the patient's medical record, the patient himself, the patient's family, and other members of the health care team.

Record your evaluation using standard terminology that all team members can easily understand and follow. For example, use the following words:

- *Continue:* No change in diagnosis, patient outcomes, or interventions is needed at this time, and the diagnosis hasn't yet been resolved.
- *Revised:* No change in diagnosis is needed, but the patient's expected outcomes and the associated interventions have been updated to reflect the patient's current status.
- *Discontinued:* A change in diagnosis is needed because additional data collection has shown that the diagnosis is no longer appropriate for the patient.
- *Achieved:* All expected outcomes have been met and the diagnosis is no longer appropriate for the patient, or one expected outcome has been met and, therefore, that portion of the care plan is marked "achieved" while the other outcomes are ongoing.
- *Reinstate:* A previous diagnosis whose outcomes had all been achieved requires renewal because the problem has recurred.

Updating the care plan

In some cases, you'll need to make modifications to the patient's care plan as a result of your evaluation. Updating typically begins with determining whether the patient has achieved the outcomes. If the outcomes haven't been fully met but your assessment shows that the problem is resolved or was inappropriately identified, the plan can be discontinued. If the problem persists, continue the plan with new outcome target dates until the desired status is achieved. If the outcomes are partially met or unmet, identify interfering factors, such as misinterpreted information or a change in the patient's status, and revise the outcomes and interventions accordingly.

When plan A doesn't work...

Updating may involve:
- clarifying or amending the database to reflect new information
- reexamining and correcting nursing diagnoses
- establishing outcome criteria that reflect new information and new or amended nursing strategies
- adding the revised nursing care plan to the original document
- recording the rationale for the revision in the progress notes.

...go to plan B...

For instance, in the case of the patient who couldn't tolerate getting out of bed to use the bathroom, even with assistance (see page 149), you could change the nursing diagnosis, patient outcome, and interventions based on the inferences you made when comparing the baseline patient data with his reassessment findings. (See *Updating a care plan.*)

...or plan C

In the event that the patient can't tolerate the activities associated with sitting on the side of the bed and, therefore, can't meet the outcome goal, revise the care plan again, beginning with your reassessment. Other nursing diagnoses that can be established based on the given findings and reassessment data may include:
- *Deficient fluid volume*
- *Risk for injury.*

Keeping priorities straight

Be sure to reprioritize the nursing diagnoses when updating your care plan. This is especially important when the patient experiences unexpected changes in his condition or possible untoward reactions as a result of his treatment or care.

Memory jogger

If you know you need to revise your patient's care plan but can't remember where to start, think **REDO:**

Reassess the patient.

Evaluate your findings.

Decide on a course of action.

Organize the care plan accordingly.

Updating a care plan

After your 78-year-old patient's experience with attempting to dangle and stand upright before walking into the bathroom, you reevaluate the established care plan. After careful reassessment, you update his care plan to include an additional nursing diagnosis and expected outcomes. One possible update is presented below:

Date	Nursing diagnosis	Expected outcomes	Interventions	Outcome evaluation (initials and date)
4/1/01	Activity intolerance related to aging process and hypovolemia as evidenced by weakness, dizziness, and increased pulse rate during activity	The patient will tolerate sitting up at the side of the bed with assistance for 10 minutes, twice per day on 7-3 shift.	• Assess functional level every shift as needed. • Obtain positional vital signs, oxygen saturation level, and pain level before starting any activity and compare these findings to morning baseline data. • Assess patient intake and output over the last 24 hours. • Monitor for signs of fatigue and avoid activity during this period. • Maintain the patient's safety. • Raise the head of the bed incrementally to reduce dizziness. • Help the patient sit on the side of the bed with the assistance of two support personnel. • Remain with the patient the entire time he's sitting upright, and assess for changes in condition or activity intolerance. • Report significant changes in the patient's condition or activity intolerance to the practitioner.	

REVIEW DATES

Date	Signature	Initials
4/1/01	Amanda Trotter	AT

When reprioritizing diagnoses, ask yourself these questions:
• Will the patient's progress be hindered if the problem isn't managed now?
• Will the patient lose functional status if the problem isn't managed now?
• Will the patient be harmed in any way that will produce a detrimental outcome if the problem isn't managed now?

A new outcome

If you're changing the nursing diagnoses, follow through by updating the expected patient outcomes (remember to include realistic, measurable goals) and specific interventions needed to achieve them. Also, make sure your interventions address any new treatments or required care (independent or collaborative) resulting from the patient's changed condition.

Last but not least

Document all of your evaluations and, as a student nurse, communicate your findings to your instructor and the patient's primary care nurse. Be sure to follow the facility's procedure for recording nurses' notes and updating nursing care plans.

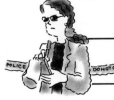

On the case

Case study background

You're assigned to care for Ella Racer, a 70 year old admitted 3 days ago with dehydration. In reviewing the admission assessment data, you note that admission vital signs were: blood pressure 90/50 mm Hg, heart rate 110 beats/minute, and respiratory rate 18 breaths/minute. Her skin color was pale and skin turgor was poor. Her weight is 145 lb (usual weight 151 lb). Initial laboratory studies indicated an elevated serum sodium level and serum osmolarity. Her care plan includes the nursing diagnosis *Deficient fluid volume related to active loss through diarrhea and inadequate intake.* Her expected outcomes are:
• The patient's fluid volume will return to normal and remain normal as evidenced by stable vital signs and a urine output at the volume established for the patient by day 3 of hospitalization.
• The patient's electrolyte values will stay within a normal range by discharge.
• The patient will express and identify three ways to prevent dehydration by discharge.
    Nursing interventions for this patient include:
• Monitor and record vital signs every 2 hours.
• Measure and record intake and output every hour. Report a urine output less than 30 ml/hour.

- Administer fluids as ordered and monitor and record effectiveness of therapy.
- Administer antidiarrheal medication as ordered.
- Weigh the patient daily at the same time.
- Monitor electrolyte levels and report abnormal values.
- Explain reasons for fluid loss and teach the patient how to avoid further episodes.

Your reassessment on day 3 reveals the following vital signs: blood pressure 110/60 mm Hg, heart rate 75 beats/minute, and respiratory rate 16 breaths/minute. Urine output is greater than 30 ml/hour. Dextrose 5% in water is infusing I.V. at 50 ml/hour. Skin color is pink and skin turgor is normal. The patient has experienced no further episodes of diarrhea and is tolerating oral fluids and solids. Electrolyte levels are within normal limits. The patient states, "I don't know how I could prevent this from happening again."

Critical thinking exercise

1. What reassessment findings show that the interventions are working?

_____

_____

_____

_____

_____

_____

2. Which interventions may no longer be necessary or could be altered?

_____

_____

_____

_____

_____

_____

3. Which of the patient's short-term goals hasn't been met?

_____

_____

_____

_____

_____

_____

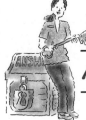

Answer key

Critical thinking exercise

1. Reassessment findings that show that interventions are working include vital signs that have returned to within normal limits (blood pressure 110/60 mm Hg, heart rate 75 beats/minute, and respiratory rate 16 breaths/minute); urine output greater than 30 ml/hour; normal skin turgor; oral fluid toleration; and electrolyte levels within normal limits.

2. Because the patient is now stable, vital signs no longer need to be taken every 2 hours. Monitoring every 4 hours or 8 hours would be adequate. Urine output could also now be measured every 4 to 8 hours.

3. Because the patient stated "I don't know how I could prevent this from happening again," the goal of "The patient will express and identify three ways to prevent dehydration by discharge" hasn't been met.

Putting it all together

Just the facts

In this chapter, you'll learn:

♦ techniques for using traditional and standardized care plans

♦ the role of computers in generating care plans

♦ components of and uses for a critical pathway

♦ types of care plans used in different health care settings.

Another look at the nursing care plan

By now, you're probably fairly well versed in the nursing process and its relationship to the nursing care plan. You know the five steps of the nursing process—assessment, nursing diagnosis, planning, implementation, and evaluation—and understand that each step builds on the previous one and that all the steps interconnect, forming the basis of a care plan.

But how does it all come together? How do you gather all the necessary information about a patient and document it correctly? And where do you, as a nursing student, fit in?

Why you need a care plan

The nursing care plan is the core of your nursing practice—a vital source of information about your patient's problems, needs, and goals and the quintessential blueprint to direct your treatment and care. When well-executed, this document can lead you step-by-step through your busy workday and help put your patient squarely on the road to wellness.

Flexible, but permanent record

Until 1991, a care plan wasn't a required part of a patient's permanent record. It may have been used by the nursing staff but, in

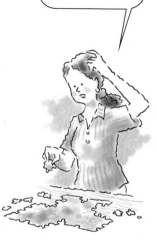

This chapter will help you put together the pieces of the care planning process.

Weighing the evidence

When did The Joint Commission become "The Boss"?

The Joint Commission (formerly the Joint Commission on Accreditation of Healthcare Organizations [JCAHO]) is often cited as the authority on standards of practice within health care organizations. However, The Joint Commission itself doesn't claim to originate standards of practice. By incorporating them into the accreditation process, the Joint Commission promotes compliance with those standards that the members of a profession have deemed essential for best practice within their specialty. This can mean engineering standards for building safety or nursing standards for excellence in provision of nursing care. The American Nurses Association and related specialty nursing organizations have determined that the nursing process, as embodied in an individualized patient care plan, is the standard of care expected of a nurse.

some facilities, it was discarded when a patient was discharged. Now, the Joint Commission mandates that the nursing care plan be permanently integrated into the medical record by paper or electronic means. (See *When did The Joint Commission become "The Boss"?*)

Joint Commission policy changes have also led to greater flexibility when writing care plans. The commission no longer specifies the format for documenting patient care, so new methods have emerged that can make planning faster and easier.

By nurses, but not just for nurses

Nursing is a unique patient-focused profession that's different from medicine and other health care fields, having its own set of diagnoses and outcomes and interventions that can be customized to meet each patient's needs. However, nurses don't work in a vacuum; they work in collaboration with other clinicians and staff to promote patient health and wellness. Consequently, although nursing care plans are developed by nurses, they may be used as a springboard to a team plan by the entire interdisciplinary team, including:

• nurses (clinical nurse specialists, registered nurses, licensed practical nurses, and nursing students)
• practitioners (physicians, physician assistants, nurse practitioners, and midwives)
• physical and occupational therapists
• speech-language pathologists
• dietitians
• respiratory therapists

The expanding world of care planning

The nursing profession isn't the only profession concerned with demonstrating the unique and crucial nature of their skills in the health care setting. Like nurses, other health care providers are seeking ways to show that their actions reflect professional accountability and represent reimbursable services from insurance companies.

Respiratory, physical, and occupational therapists; registered dietitians; speech-language pathologists; and nutritional specialists all assess patients, analyze their findings, develop treatment plans, implement their plans, and reassess the effectiveness of their plans. The standards of practice for these professionals make it clear that these are mandated functions.

In many long-term care facilities, assisted-living facilities, inpatient psychiatric centers, and home care and hospice agencies, these professionals are active members of an interdisciplinary team that develops an overall care plan for each patient. As such, a dietitian might collaborate with nursing staff to include specific interventions in the nursing care plan that promote certain outcomes—for example, obtaining optimal nutrition or skin integrity. A physical or occupational therapist might be involved in developing some of the nursing interventions for a patient with a diagnosis of *Impaired physical mobility.* Depending on the facility, these specialists may document their assessment findings and care on an interdisciplinary form or their own standard forms.

- social workers and discharge planners
- pharmacists
- clergy.

All on the same team

Each member of the interdisciplinary team may have some input in developing the care plan, but the registered nurse is responsible for making sure that it's carried out on a daily basis and documented according to the facility's policies. Other team members can also document their interventions on the care plan under their specified column or box. (See *The expanding world of care planning.*)

Students' role in care planning

As a student, you should read and be knowledgeable about your patient's care plan at the hospital, nursing home, or agency where you perform clinical rounds. Each facility and department oper-

Teacher knows best

Paper trail

As you proceed through your clinical rotations, the type of paperwork you're required to complete might change. An early focus may be on the nursing assessment and correlating those findings with the medical history and diagnosis. Later, you may be required to complete medication work-sheets that focus on helping you learn about hundreds of drugs and what to teach the patients taking them. Finally come the nursing care plans themselves, in various formats and detail. All of these tools serve one essential purpose: to widen your knowledge base and sharpen your thinking skills so you can make decisions logically and quickly as you care for patients.

ates differently, so it's your responsibility to become familiar with the system used.

RN recording rights

Keep in mind that only registered nurses can create and update a nursing care plan. In some institutions, licensed practical nurses can assist with writing the care plan, but they're only permitted to do so under the supervision of a registered nurse. The registered nurse remains the one accountable for the correctness, implementation, and evaluation of the plan and is the only team member permitted to change the nursing portions of the plan.

Student's right to write

As a student, you may use and follow the established care plan, but you can't document on it. You'll document your patient findings, nursing care, and observations directly on the medication records, flow sheets, treatment plans, and progress notes. However, you're expected to create your own care plan or concept map to use during clinical rotations. Even when you don't have to turn a written care plan in to your instructor, you're accountable for having developed a care plan for the day and being able to verbalize it to your instructor when asked. (See *Paper trail.*)

Types of care plans

Care plans are usually written in one of two styles: traditional or standardized. As a student or a newly graduated nurse, you're more likely to see and use standardized care plans; in most cases, they're easier to use and they're more common than traditional plans. Another issue is the increasing use of electronic health records systems that include a care planning function. These systems are a variation on standardized care plans but require some special mention. Regardless of which type you use, your care plan should cover all aspects of nursing care, from admission to discharge.

Traditional care plans

Also called an *individually developed plan*, a traditional care plan is written to your patient's specific problems and causative factors. After you analyze your assessment data for a patient, you either write the plan by hand or enter it into a computer. (See *Traditional, but highly personalized*, page 164.)

Home-baked from scratch

The basic form for the traditional care plan varies, depending on the function of this important document in your facility or department. Most forms have four main columns:

- nursing diagnoses
- expected outcomes
- interventions
- outcome evaluations.

The form may also have columns for the date when you initiated the care plan, target dates for expected outcomes, and the dates for review, revisions, and resolutions. Most forms also have a place for you to sign or initial whenever you make an entry or revision.

Looking toward an outcome

The information that you should include on a traditional care plan form varies, too. Because shorter hospital stays are more common today, in some facilities, you're expected to write only short-term outcomes that the patient can reach by the time he's discharged. However, other facilities—especially long-term care facilities—may also want you to chart long-term outcomes for the patient's maximum functioning level. These facilities commonly provide forms with separate spaces for short-term and long-term outcomes.

Personal, visual, clear

The traditional method has several advantages:
- It provides a personalized plan for each patient.

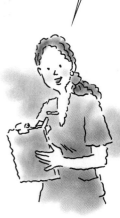

Traditional care plans can be written by hand or entered into a computer.

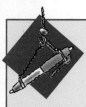

Under construction

Traditional, but highly personalized

Here's an example of a traditional care plan. It shows how these forms are typically organized. Remember that a traditional plan is written from scratch for each patient. These types of plans are becoming less common with the advent of electronic products containing modifiable standardized care plans.

Date	Nursing diagnosis	Expected outcomes	Interventions	Outcome evaluation (initials and date)
6/21/01	Ineffective breathing pattern R/T pain as evidenced by c/o pain with deep breaths or coughing and shallow respirations at 22 to 26 breaths/minute	The patient will maintain respiratory rate of 16 to 20 breaths/minute with normal depth while awake within 8 hours and ongoing.	• Assess and record respiratory status, including pulse oximetry q4h. • Assess for pain q3h and 1 hour after each dosage of pain medication. • Give pain medication as ordered p.r.n. • Assist patient to comfortable position q2h while awake. • Teach patient how, when, and why to use incentive spirometer.	*Nursing diagnoses, expected outcomes, interventions, and outcome evaluations are key elements of traditional care plans.*
		The patient will rate pain as 3 or less on a 0-to-10 scale while using an incentive spirometer 10 times hourly while awake within 4 hours and ongoing.	• Demonstrate to patient how to splint chest while coughing. • Encourage patient to use spirometer 10 times/hour while awake as long as bedrest is maintained. • Provide rest periods between care activities. • Initiate oxygen therapy as ordered per given parameters.	

REVIEW DATES

Date	Signature	Initials
6/28/01	C. Planner, RN	CP

- The format allows health care team members and the patient to easily visualize the plan.
- Columns for outcome evaluations are clearly delineated.

Time isn't on its side

The main disadvantage of a traditional plan is that it's time-consuming to read and write because it requires lengthy documentation.

Standardized care plans

Standardized care plans are more commonly used. They eliminate the problems associated with traditional plans by using preprinted information. This saves documentation time. (See *Standardized saves time*, page 166.)

Some standardized plans are classified by medical diagnoses or diagnosis-related groups (DRGs); others, by nursing diagnoses. The preprinted information included in a standardized care plan includes interventions for patients with similar diagnoses and, usually, root outcome statements.

Insist on individuality

Early versions of standardized care plans didn't allow for differences in patients' needs. However, current versions require you to explain how you have individualized the plan for each patient by adding the following information:
• "related to" (R/T) statements and signs and symptoms for a nursing diagnosis—If the form provides a root diagnosis, such as "Acute pain R/T _____," you might fill in *inflammation, as exhibited by grimacing and other expressions of pain.*
• time limits for the outcomes—To a root statement of the goal *Perform postural drainage without assistance,* you might add *for 15 minutes immediately upon awakening in the morning by 11/12.*
• frequency of interventions—To an intervention, such as *Perform passive range-of-motion exercises,* you might add *twice per day: in the morning and in the evening.*
• specific instruction for interventions—For the standard intervention *Elevate the patient's head,* you might specify *before sleep, on three pillows.*

Computers make combos less cumbersome

When a patient has more than one diagnosis, you must use all the standardized care plans, which can make records long and cumbersome. However, if your facility uses computerized standard care plans, you may be able to extract only the parts you need for each plan and then combine them to make one manageable plan. Some computer programs provide a checklist of interventions from which you can select to build your own plans.

> Standardized care plans are commonly completed on a computer.

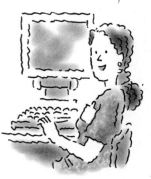

Standardized saves time

A standardized care plan can save you valuable time. The plan below is for a patient with a nursing diagnosis of *Impaired tissue integrity*. To customize this standardized care plan to one of your patients, you would complete the diagnosis—including signs and symptoms—and fill in the expected outcomes.

Date 4/15/01

Nursing diagnosis
Impaired tissue integrity *Related to arterial insufficiency as evidenced by pain in calves and pressure area with walking; stage 2 ulcer on ⓡ fourth toe, bilateral +1 nonpitting edema, cool temperature, and sluggish capillary circulation in right foot*

Target date
    4/17/01
    4/17/01
    4/17/01

    4/19/01

Expected outcomes
Attains relief from immediate symptoms: *Pain and edema will resolve*
Voices intent to change tissue aggravating behavior: *Will stop smoking immediately*
Maintains collateral circulation: *Palpable peripheral pulses in lower extremities, extremities warm*
Voices intent to follow specific management routines after discharge: *Foot-care guidelines, exercise regimen as specified by physical therapist*

Date 4/15/01

Interventions
• Provide foot and ulcer care. Administer and monitor treatments according to facility protocols.
• Encourage adherence to an exercise regimen as tolerated.
• Educate the patient about risk factors and injury prevention measures. Refer the patient to a stop-smoking program on discharge.
• Maintain adequate hydration. Monitor I/O: *q8 hours*
• Elevate the head of bed: *6" to 8"*
• Additional interventions: *Inspect skin integrity q6h; assess peripheral pulses, skin temperature and color, and capillary refill q8h; administer analgesics before ulcer care and physical therapy as ordered p.r.n.*

Date
    4/17/01

    4/17/01

    4/17/01

    4/17/01

Outcome evaluation
Attained relief of immediate symptoms: *Pain and edema resolved, stage 2 ulcer continues; outcome partially met, extend expected outcome to 4/19/01 or discharge if earlier*
Voiced intent to change tissue aggravating behavior: *Hasn't smoked since admission, verbalizes desire to remain nonsmoking after discharge with help of nicotine patch or gum if needed; outcome met*
Maintained collateral circulation: *Palpable peripheral pulses bilaterally, right diminished compared to left; right lower extremity cooler to touch than left; capillary refill sluggish but equal bilaterally; outcome partially met, extend expected outcome to 4/19/01 or discharge if earlier*
Voiced intent to follow specific management routines after discharge: *Verbalizes understanding of foot-care and exercise guidelines given, and willingness to continue regimen after discharge; outcome met*

Although standardized plans usually include only essential information, most provide space for you to write additional expected outcomes, interventions, and outcome evaluations.

The pros

Standardized care plans offer many advantages because they:
• require far less writing than traditional plans
• are more legible
• are easier to duplicate
• make compliance with a facility's policy easier for all members of the health care team, including experts, novices, and ancillary staff
• guide you in creating the plan and allow you the freedom to adapt it to your patient.

The cons (there's always at least one)

This method has one main drawback: If you simply check off items on a list or fill in the blanks, you might not individualize the patient's care or document your findings adequately.

Computerized care plans

In the health care industry, the first area of extensive conversion to electronics was institutional accounting. However, in the past 10 years, the push has been toward integrating accounting systems with a complete electronic health record (EHR). Today, you're increasingly likely to encounter computerized care plans during your clinical rotations.

Different strokes for different folks

Various types of software are available for different facility needs. Some systems are programmed to generate a list of nursing diagnoses after the patient's assessment data is entered. You can modify the selected items as needed. Others require you to choose the diagnoses yourself from a master list. The system then adds these diagnoses to the patient's EHR.

EHRs also offer different styles of care planning. Some systems rely on generalized care plans written to a patient problem or profile, not to a specific nursing diagnosis. For example, in the sample electronic shift report shown on page 125, note that the patient's care plan was called "General care of the adult" and included two nursing protocols (Falls prevention and Skin breakdown [prevention]), plus a Clinical guideline (CVA). A very general goal is listed: "Patient will tolerate a progressive increase in activity level." However, some EHR products are moving toward integrating the taxonomies of NANDA International, Nursing Interventions Classification, and Nursing Outcomes Classification into the process.

RN input

Like traditional and standardized plans, a computerized care plan must be reviewed by a registered nurse every 24 hours. Remember that despite their efficiency and ability to access information quickly, computer software systems can't replace a nurse's critical thinking and decision-making skills. Nurses still have to decide which diagnoses and interventions are most appropriate for any given patient and must evaluate when changes to the care plan are needed.

Care plans in different settings

As you begin your clinical rotations, you'll notice that different units and care settings sometimes use different care plan formats. For example, acute care units, including psychiatric centers, commonly use standardized care plans or critical pathways. Same-day surgery units often use a problem-list format rather than an actual care plan, but it serves the same purpose.

Have diagnosis, will travel

The standardized care plans available on each unit are usually selected to fit the type of patient medical diagnoses common to the unit. For example, a medical-surgical unit might have different standard plans than the maternity or psychiatric unit. However, a resource containing all plans should be available to all staff because patients may have more than one diagnosis, some of which may not be included in the standardized plans for the patient's assigned unit. For example, a patient on a psychiatric unit may have coexisting nursing diagnoses related to an ongoing medical diagnosis, such as diabetes or gastroesophageal reflux disease. Conversely, a patient with schizophrenia may be admitted to an oncology unit for treatment of cancer. Holistic patient care requires attention to all diagnoses because each impacts the patient's healing capacity.

Acute care hospital units

On most acute care units, care plans are separate documents that are formulated at the time of a patient's admission (typically within the first 8 hours). Although nursing interventions begin immediately with a patient's admission, the care plan takes careful plan-

> Note that different care settings use different types of care plans.

ning and collaborative input and serves as a legal document of the care being given.

Most facilities require that care plans be reviewed and updated by a registered nurse at least every 24 hours, beginning with the time of admission. Accreditation organizations, such as the Joint Commission, perform spot-checks of individual patient charts to see whether a care plan is present and if it was reviewed within the established time-frame.

Fill in the blanks...

Some units use preprinted plans on which the nursing diagnosis is already written; the nurse fills in a "related to" clause as well as in-dividualized interventions, making the care plan specific to the pa-tient. For example, for a patient with a nursing diagnosis of *Acute pain*, the nurse might fill in *related to surgical procedure* or *relat-ed to pneumonia with pleural effusion*, depending on the reason for the pain. The interventions, of course, would be filled in based on the patient's needs and circumstances.

...or check 'em off

Other units use preprinted care plans that include a comprehen-sive list of interventions. In this case, the nurse simply checks off the interventions applicable to her patient's problem.

Multiple problems

Usually, patients on medical-surgical units have multiple nursing diagnoses that must be addressed. All of the diagnoses for one pa-tient are considered one care plan. For example, a patient admit-ted with a fractured left tibia might have the following diagnoses:
* *Acute pain related to compound fracture of tibia*
* *Risk for infection related to multiple breaks in skin integrity of left leg*
* *Impaired physical mobility related to fractured left tibia as evidenced by inability to bear weight on left leg and X-rays showing compound fracture.*

Keeping priorities straight

Within the care plan, the nursing diagnoses must be prioritized ac-cording to the level of importance for the patient. For example, suppose you've assessed a patient admitted with acute heart fail-ure and have identified these diagnoses:
* *Excess fluid volume related to sodium and water retention*
* *Activity intolerance related to shortness of breath and fatigue*
* *Decreased cardiac output related to impaired contractility*
* *Impaired urinary elimination (hesitancy) related to benign prostate enlargement*

- *Ineffective tissue perfusion (cardiopulmonary, peripheral) related to decreased cardiac output*
- *Anxiety related to acute increase in shortness of breath.*

You might prioritize these nursing diagnoses as follows:
- *Decreased cardiac output*
- *Excess fluid volume*
- *Ineffective tissue perfusion*
- *Anxiety*
- *Impaired urinary elimination*
- *Activity intolerance.*

Take the critical pathway

A critical pathway is a special type of care plan that's used by the interdisciplinary team, not just nurses, so it's more collaborative in nature. It includes assessment criteria, interventions, treatments, and outcomes for specific conditions according to a time line that's based on an average patient's expected length of stay. Actual time-frames can be modified to meet each patient's needs.

Complete coverage

Think of a critical pathway as a predetermined checklist describing the tasks you and the patient must accomplish. Unlike a nursing care plan, its focus is interdisciplinary, covering all of the patient's problems, not just those identified during a nursing assessment. For example, it may include specific interventions for physical assessment, lab work and procedures, consultations, medication administration, nutrition, elimination, activity and therapy, patient teaching, and discharge planning. (See *Using a critical pathway*, pages 172 and 173.)

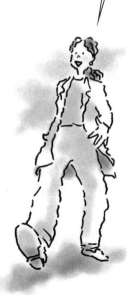

> Think of a critical pathway as a predetermined checklist that describes the steps you and the patient must take.

Same-day surgery unit

On a same-day surgery unit, nurses may follow an abbreviated standardized plan that addresses the patient's specific type of surgery or procedure. Additional medical diagnoses are listed and interventions are added related to those diagnoses if needed. The nurse typically reviews the problem list before and after the surgery or procedure. If the patient requires admittance to the hospital, a full nursing care plan is developed, using the problem list as a starting point.

Extended-care facilities

Nursing homes and other extended-care facilities have a different system for formulating care plans. Most of these facilities provide services for individuals who qualify for Medicare or Medicaid insurance benefits due to their age or severe disability. Medicare regulations have become the standard of care for extended-care facilities so that even private insurers look for verification that a facility meets these standards. Part of these standards requires the completion of the Minimum Data Set (MDS) form, which documents patient assessment and care screening and guides reimbursement levels. Each facility employs a registered nurse as the RN Assessment Coordinator (RNAC). This person is responsible for completing and submitting the MDS and other required forms and running the weekly interdisciplinary team meetings at which care plans are finalized and reviewed for each resident. The RNAC meets with residents and their families, communicates with all staff members involved in the resident's care, and reviews all documentation to verify that required information has been completed.

Mirror, mirror on the wall

If you have a chance to do a clinical rotation in an extended-care facility, you may find that this setting most closely mirrors the use of the nursing process and nursing and interdisciplinary care planning as you have been taught in school. Because residents have chronic conditions requiring 24-hour care, nursing diagnoses may be relevant for long time periods. Expected outcomes tend to focus less on healing and resumption of prior function than on maintaining the present level of function and developing skills to adapt to limitations in function. However, always be alert for those situations where a rehabilitative goal is appropriate, such as fractured bones, episodic lung or urinary infections, situational depression or anxiety disorders, or new urinary incontinence issues.

Don't break the rules

An RNAC has up to 7 days to complete the MDS and 14 days to develop an individualized care plan for each new resident. In the meantime, a generic care plan must be initiated within 24 hours. Common nursing diagnoses in extended care facilities include:
- *Chronic pain*
- *Risk for injury*
- *Activity intolerance*
- *Risk for infection*
- *Risk for impaired skin integrity*
- *Impaired environmental interpretation syndrome.*

Each resident must have a complete reassessment yearly, including a complete physical examination by a physician. Guidelines have been set for frequency of documentation by each discipline, review of the medical orders, and evaluation and updating of the interdisciplinary care plan.

(Text continues on page 174.)

Using a critical pathway

At any point in a patient's treatment, a glance at the critical pathway allows you to compare the patient's progress and your performance as a caregiver with the usual course of care and progress for other patients with the same diagnosis. Critical pathways are based on analytical studies as well as the standards of care established by the professional group most closely allied with treatment of the disorder.

Example

The standard critical pathway below outlines care for a patient with a colon resection.

CRITICAL PATHWAY: COLON RESECTION WITHOUT COLOSTOMY				
	Patient visit	**Presurgery day 1**	**Day 0 O.R. day**	**Postoperative day 1**
Assessments	History and physical with breast, rectal, and pelvic examinations Nursing assessment	Nursing admission assessment	Nursing admission assessment on TBA patients in holding area Postoperative review of systems assessment*	Review of systems assessment*
Consults	Social service consult Physical therapy consult	Notify referring doctor of impending admission		
Labs and diagnostics	Complete blood count (CBC) PT/PTT Electrocardiogram Chest X-ray (CXR) Chemistry profile CT scan ABD w/wo contrast CT scan pelvis Urinalysis Barium enema and flexible sigmoidoscopy or colonoscopy Biopsy report	Type and screen for patients with Hg level < 10	Type and screen for patients in holding area with Hg level < 10	CB⟨
Interventions	Many or all of the above labs and diagnostics will have already been done. Check all results and fax to the surgeon's	Admit by 0800 Check for bowel preparation orders Bowel preparation* Antiembolism stockings Incentive spirometry Ankle exercises* I.V. access* Routine VS* Pneumatic inflation boots	Shave and prepare in operating room NG tube maintenance* I/O VS per routine* Foley care* Incentive spirometry* Ankle exercises* I.V. site care* HOB 30° Safety measures* Wound care* Mouth care*	NG tube maintenance* I/O* VS per routine* Foley care* Incentive spirometry* Ankle exercises* I.V. site care* HOB 30°* Safety measures* Wound care* Mouth care* Antiembolism stockings
I.V.s		I.V. fluids, $D_5\frac{1}{2}$ NSS	I.V. fluids, D_5LR	I.V. fluids, D₅LR
Medication	Prescribe GoLYTELY or NuLYTELY 1000-1400 Neomycin @ 1400, 1500, and 2200 Erythromycin @ 1400, 1500, and 2200	GoLYTELY or NuLYTELY 1000-1400 Erythromycin @ 1400, 1500, and 2200 Neomycin @ 1400, 1500, and 2200	Preoperative ABX in holding area Postoperative ABX × 2 doses PCA (basal rate 0.5 mg) subQ heparin	
Diet/GI	Clears presurgery day NPO after midnight	Clears presurgery day NPO after midnight	NPO/NG tube	
Activity			4 hours after surgery ambulate with abdominal binder* D/C pneumatic inflation boots after patient ambulates	Ambulate t.i.d. with abdominal binder* May shower Physical therapy b.i.d.
KEY: * = NSG Activities **V = Variance** **N = No Variance**	1. 2. 3. V V V Ⓝ N N	1. 2. 3. V V V Ⓝ Ⓝ Ⓝ	1. 2. 3. V V V Ⓝ Ⓝ Ⓝ	1. 2. 3. V V V Ⓝ Ⓝ Ⓝ
Signatures:	1. _C. Malloy, RN_ 2. _____ 3. _____	1. _M Connel, RN_ 2. _J. Smith, RN_ 3. _P. Joseph, RN_	1. _L. Singer, RN_ 2. _J. Smith, RN_ 3. _P. Joseph, RN_	1. _L. Singer, RN_ 2. _J. Smith, RN_ 3. _P. Joseph, RN_

> The pathway designates a specific time frame for patient care activities.

> The pathway is organized into categories based on the patient's medical diagnosis.

> The pathway lists tasks that the patient and caregivers need to accomplish.

CRITICAL PATHWAY: COLON RESECTION WITHOUT COLOSTOMY

	Postoperative day 2	Postoperative day 3	Postoperative day 4	Postoperative day 5
Assessments	Review of systems assessment*	Review of systems assessment*	Review of systems assessment*	Review of systems assessment*
Consults		Dietary consult		Oncology consult if indicated (Dukes B2 or C or high-risk lesion) (or to be done as outpatient)
Labs and diagnostics	Electrolyte 7 (EL-7) CXR	CBC EL-7	Pathology results on chart	CBC EL-7
Interventions	Discontinue NG tube if possible* (per guidelines) I/O* VS per routine* Discontinue Foley* Ambulating* Incentive spirometry* Ankle exercises* I.V. site care* HOB 30°* Safety measures* Wound care* Mouth care* Antiembolism stockings	I/O* VS per routine* Incentive spirometry* Ankle exercises* I.V. site care* Safety measures* Wound care* Antiembolism stockings	I/O* VS per routine* Incentive spirometry* Ankle exercises* I.V. site care* Safety measures* Wound care* Antiembolism stockings	Consider staple removal Replace with Steri-Strips Assess that patient has met discharge criteria* Discontinue saline lock
I.V.s	I.V. fluids D₅½ NSS+ MVI	I.V. convert to saline lock	Continue saline lock	Disco[...]
Medication	PCA (0.5 mg basal rate)	Discontinue PCA P.O. analgesia Resume routine home meds	P.O. analgesia Preoperative meds	P.O. analgesia Preoperative meds
Diet/GI	Discontinue NG tube per guidelines: (Clamp tube at 8 a.m. if no N/V and residual < 200 ml, D/C tube @ 1200)* (Check with doctor first)	Clears if+bm/flatus Advance to postoperative diet if tolerating clears (at least one tray of clears)	House	House
Activity	Ambulate q.i.d. with abdominal binder* May shower Physical therapy b.i.d.	Ambulate at least q.i.d. with abdominal binder* May shower Physical therapy b.i.d.	Ambulate at least q.i.d. with abdominal binder* May shower Physical therapy b.i.d.	
Teaching	Reinforce preoperative teaching* Patient and family education p.r.n.* Re: family screening	Reinforce preoperative teaching* Patient and family education p.r.n.* Re: family screening Begin discharge teaching	Reinforce preoperative teaching* Patient and family education p.r.n.* Discharge teaching re: reportable s/s, follow-up, and wound care*	Review all discharge instructions and Rx including:* follow-up appointments: with surgeon within 3 weeks with oncologist within 1 month if indicated
KEY: * = NSG Activities V = Variance N = No Var.	1. V Ⓝ 2. V Ⓝ 3. V Ⓝ	1. V Ⓝ 2. V Ⓝ 3. V Ⓝ	1. V Ⓝ 2. V Ⓝ 3. V Ⓝ	1. V Ⓝ 2. V Ⓝ 3. V N
Signatures:	1. _A. McCarthy, RN_ 2. _R. Moyer, RN_ 3. _L. Waters, RN_	1. _A. McCarthy, RN_ 2. _R. Moyer, RN_ 3. _L. Waters, RN_	1. _L. Singer, RN_ 2. _J. Smith, RN_ 3. _P. Joseph, RN_	1. _L. Singer, RN_ 2. _J. Smith, RN_ 3.

The pathway lists key events that must occur before the patient's discharge date.

Hospice care

Hospice programs also use care plans for their patients. In this setting, the care plan is prepared by an interdisciplinary team comprised of nurses, certified nursing assistants, physicians, therapists, clergy, volunteers, bereavement counselors, and social workers. It's reviewed daily and updated every 2 weeks. (For inpatient hospice patients, care plans may be reviewed on a weekly basis.) All hospice programs, regardless of the setting, must follow Medicare rules and regulations if they wish to accept patients under the Medicare hospice benefit program.

Creating care plans: A summary

As previously discussed, everything you do as a nurse focuses on the nursing process, and care plans are a natural extension of that process. Your patient's care plan is a summary of his problems, his goals, and the care he receives. It's also your key to helping him achieve wellness.

Revisiting the nursing process

You'll start developing your care plan beginning with your patient's initial assessment. This is when you'll talk with the patient and his family members to gather subjective and objective data, perform a physical examination, and obtain the medical history.

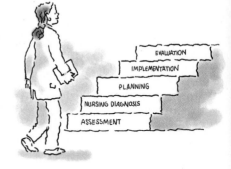

Taking it step by step

From all this information, you'll develop your nursing diagnoses, collaborate with the patient to identify his outcome goals, and begin planning interventions to achieve those goals. The plan you come up with—the nursing care plan—directs your patient care from that moment forward.

Why you do what you do

As a student, remember to include a rationale (reason) and cite the reference source, as appropriate, for each intervention. The rationale is the "why" behind the "what."

Why is it necessary to ambulate a surgical patient on the first postoperative day? Why should you assess lung sounds every 4 hours if your patient has heart failure? Right now, you're learning the answers to these and other questions in your classroom setting and by researching journals and other textbooks. With each new patient, you'll acquire more and more knowledge and hone your critical thinking skills. Soon such questions, and their corresponding rationales, will become second nature to you.

As a practicing nurse, you won't include rationales in the patient's care plan. But don't think this lets you off the hook! Nursing is continually evolving, just like medicine in general. Long-trusted techniques and standards of care may be rejected as research shows better ways to accomplish the same tasks. Throughout your career, you'll need to stay up-to-date with the latest evidence-based practice and standards of care. In fact, many states require registered nurses to have several continuing-education credits to renew their nursing licenses.

Evaluating and reassessing at every turn

Keep in mind that, as you perform each intervention, you'll need to evaluate your patient's condition and response to the intervention. In some cases, these responses will require you to change the care plan accordingly. For example, your patient may not be able to walk the distance specified in his care plan or his pneumonia may be clearing up and you won't need to assess his breath sounds as frequently as specified in the care plan. Such changes mean reexamining the interventions and expected outcome and making necessary modifications if the patient hasn't yet achieved his outcome goal.

Sample care plans and concept maps

During your rotations, you'll probably care for patients in maternity, pediatric, psychiatric, and medical-surgical settings. On the pages that follow, you'll find sample patient scenarios, with corresponding concept maps and care plans, for some of these settings. These care plans and concept maps are included to help you analyze how a care plan comes together. As you review these sample plans, try to think of other possible diagnoses, outcomes, and interventions that might be appropriate for these patients.

Welcome, Baby!

An 18-year-old female, Patricia Thomas, just gave birth to an 8 lb, 2 oz baby boy via cesarean delivery. She isn't married, but her boyfriend is present. Her parents are also present but are visibly tense. The patient's vital signs are stable, but she's in pain. She states that she wants to breast-feed the baby, so you assist her in turning on her side and you position the baby beside her. You show her how to get the baby to latch on, but the young mother is having difficulty and becomes frustrated. "Don't give up," says the boyfriend.

This patient's care plan focuses on the nursing diagnoses *Deficient knowledge (breast-feeding)* and *Acute pain*. The concept map for this patient might look like this:

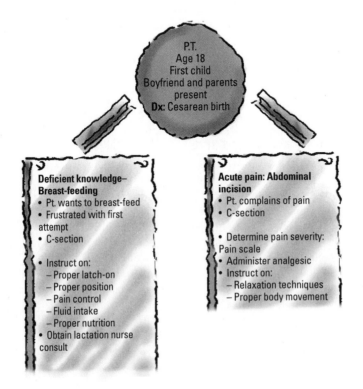

See *Sample maternal-neonatal care plan* to see what the care plan might look like.

Sample maternal-neonatal care plan

Here's an example of what the care plan might look like for the maternal patient described in the text.

Nursing diagnosis 1
Deficient knowledge (breast-feeding) related to being a young, first-time mother who's new to breast-feeding

Outcome
The mother will demonstrate proper latching on technique and nursing positions before discharge. The baby will have a good suck reflex and audible swallowing.

Interventions	Rationale
1. Teach the mother proper latch-on technique.	1. Proper latch-on ensures proper sucking by infant, which in turn affects milk supply.
2. Instruct the mother on the different nursing positions, especially the side-lying and football-hold positions, which are best for post-cesarean-delivery patients.	2. Positioning to decrease strain on the incision and increase neonatal comfort and safety is conducive to let-down.
3. Offer and administer pain medications as needed.	3. Being pain-free helps the mother relax and promotes the let-down reflex.
4. Encourage the mother to drink at least 8 glasses of fluid per day.	4. Good hydration is essential for a healthy milk supply.
5. Encourage the mother to increase her caloric intake.	5. Breast-feeding moms need to consume 500 calories more per day than they did when they were pregnant to help with milk production.
6. Obtain an order for a lactation nurse if needed.	6. Lactation nurses specialize in dealing with breast-feeding problems and offering correct information.

(continued)

Sample maternal-neonatal care plan *(continued)*

Nursing diagnosis 2
Acute pain related to abdominal incision from cesarean delivery as evidenced by verbalization of pain and slowed movements in and out of bed

Outcome
The mother will verbalize decreased pain each day and minimal pain by discharge.

Interventions	Rationale
1. Assess and document severity of pain every shift and as needed, using a 0-to-10 pain scale.	1. Knowing the patient's pain severity assists in providing the correct type and dose of pain medication.
2. Administer pain medication as ordered.	2. Pain medications help alleviate pain and promote rest.
3. Teach the mother not to wait for pain to get severe before asking for pain medication.	3. Severe pain may require more medication or more time to become alleviated.
4. Teach the mother relaxation techniques.	4. Relaxation techniques help lessen pain perception and can assist with coping with stress at home.
5. Teach the mother the proper techniques for getting out of a chair and bed.	5. Proper movements help minimize discomfort and pain when getting up.

Feeling the blues

A 65-year-old female, Julie Blue, is admitted with depression and inadequate nutrition due to lack of eating. Her husband of 45 years passed away unexpectedly 1 year ago, and she hasn't been coping well with his death. Her daughter brought her to the hospital because she couldn't get her mother to eat, bathe, get out of bed, or brush her hair for 2 weeks.

The patient states, "I just can't go on without my husband. He did everything." The daughter also tells the nurse that the electric and water have been turned off because her mother keeps forgetting to pay the bills.

The concept map for this patient might look like this:

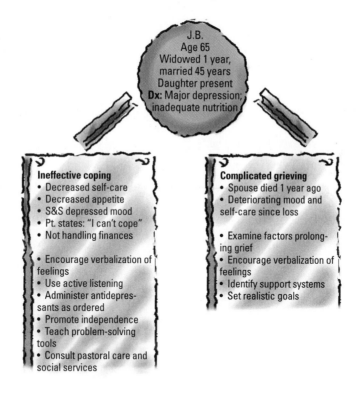

J.B.
Age 65
Widowed 1 year,
married 45 years
Daughter present
Dx: Major depression;
inadequate nutrition

Ineffective coping
• Decreased self-care
• Decreased appetite
• S&S depressed mood
• Pt. states: "I can't cope"
• Not handling finances

• Encourage verbalization of feelings
• Use active listening
• Administer antidepressants as ordered
• Promote independence
• Teach problem-solving tools
• Consult pastoral care and social services

Complicated grieving
• Spouse died 1 year ago
• Deteriorating mood and self-care since loss

• Examine factors prolonging grief
• Encourage verbalization of feelings
• Identify support systems
• Set realistic goals

See *Sample psychiatric care plan*, pages 180 and 181, to see what the care plan might look like.

Sample psychiatric care plan

Here's an example of what the care plan might look like for the patient described in the text.

Nursing diagnosis 1

Ineffective coping related to sudden death of spouse 1 year ago as evidenced by lack of self-care and verbalization of inability to cope

Outcome

The patient will verbalize feelings about the death of her husband and demonstrate new coping mechanisms by discharge.

Interventions	Rationale
1. Encourage the patient to talk about her feelings.	1. Verbalizing feelings makes the patient and others aware of what the patient is going through.
2. Use active listening and a calm, unhurried manner.	2. This approach conveys to the patient your concern and willingness to listen.
3. Administer antidepressants as ordered.	3. Medications may be essential to assist the patient with the mood disorder.
4. Encourage the patient to independently perform at least one activity of daily living each day.	4. Self-care helps improve patient outlook, self-worth, and independence.
5. Teach the patient problem-solving tools, such as the step-by-step approach and weighing advantages and disadvantages.	5. Knowledge of problem-solving tools assists with day-to-day activities on discharge.
6. Allow the patient time to solve at least one simple problem per day on her own (such as what to eat or wear).	6. Successful problem solving promotes independence and self-confidence.
7. Assist the patient in identifying problems or issues that she can't control or change.	7. Helping the patient realize her limitations decreases stress and feelings of incompetence.
8. Obtain an order for consults with pastoral care and social services, as needed.	8. Spiritual guidance or assistance with other issues may be helpful as the patient identifies issues of concern.

Sample psychiatric care plan (continued)

Nursing diagnosis 2
Complicated grieving related to loss of spouse as evidenced by depression, social isolation, inability to cope with ADLs

Outcome
The patient will verbalize feelings of grief and demonstrate use of new coping methods for managing her feelings by discharge.

Interventions	Rationale
1. Assess for factors that are prolonging the grieving process.	1. Identifying a problem will help to solve it.
2. Encourage the patient to talk about feelings of grief, anger, and depression in individual and group therapy sessions.	2. Acknowledging feelings is first step to finding ways to deal with them.
3. Assist the patient in identifying her support systems.	3. Support systems can help patient in time of emotional need.
4. Discuss with the patient methods to cope with stresses such as focusing on living life "one day at a time."	4. Planning too far ahead can increase stress as new coping skills are developed.
5. Assist the patient in setting realistic goals.	5. Accomplishing short term goals will help her gain a sense of control of her life.

Boy, oh boy!

A 10-year-old boy with cystic fibrosis, Bobby Young, is admitted to the hospital with upper respiratory infection and fever. His oral temperature is 101.6° F. He's coughing up copious amounts of yellowish green sputum. He's talkative but tires easily. His mother says his symptoms started about 2 days ago; she noticed that he'd gone to bed earlier because he was tired and that he appeared to be coughing more in the evening. She gave him an extra breathing treatment last night, but it didn't seem to help. The patient has been drinking his fluids well and taking his medications without any problems. His lung sounds on admission reveal rhonchi throughout the lower lobes. He has no acute shortness of breath and no other problems. His chest X-ray reveals no significant findings.

The concept map for this patient might look like this:

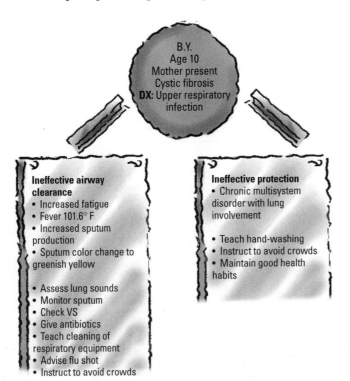

See *Sample pediatric care plan* to see what the care plan might look like. Note that this care plan addresses the patient's present infection and ongoing infection risk.

And many more...

Throughout your nursing career, you're likely to create or encounter plenty of nursing care plans. Using the previous examples, and everything you've learned about care planning in this book, see if you can create your own care plan for the medical-surgical patient described in the *On the case* quiz on page 184.

Sample pediatric care plan

Here's an example of what the care plan might look like for the patient described in the text.

Nursing diagnosis 1

Ineffective airway clearance related to acute respiratory infection as evidenced by increased amount of sputum, yellow-green sputum color, increased fatigue, and fever

Outcome

The patient will demonstrate clear lung sounds, lack of fever, and return to baseline energy level by discharge.

Interventions	Rationale
1. Assess lungs sounds and respiratory pattern every shift and as needed.	1. Early recognition of worsening condition leads to early treatment and improved patient outcomes.
2. Assess amount, color, and consistency of sputum every shift.	2. Increased amounts, thickening, and continued color change of sputum can indicate worsening infection.
3. Assess vital signs every shift. Report deteriorating findings to the practitioner.	3. Increasing temperature and respirations indicate poor response to treatment.
4. Administer antibiotics as ordered.	4. Antibiotics help to fight infection.
5. Teach the patient and family proper cleaning of respiratory equipment.	5. Proper cleaning of respiratory equipment helps to prevent bacterial growth.
6. Teach the patient the importance of avoiding crowds during flu season and getting a flu shot.	6. Cystic fibrosis puts the patient at higher risk for infection. Avoiding crowds limits exposure to the flu. Getting a flu shot provides additional protection.

Nursing diagnosis 2

Ineffective protection related to cystic fibrosis as evidenced by ongoing sputum production, enzymatic disorder, and increased risk of infection

Outcome

The patient and family will verbalize understanding of instructions on risk reduction by discharge.

Interventions	Rationale
1. Reinforce with the patient and family that proactive hand washing is a major defense against secondary infection.	1. Hand washing prevents incidental exposure to infection.
2. Teach the patient and family to actively avoid crowded environments during flu season and to avoid people who are ill.	2. Active attention to environmental risks can decrease exposure to infectious agents.
3. Teach the patient to maintain healthy rest, nutrition, and lung maintenance programs.	3. Healthy daily habits promote increased resistance to infectious agents.

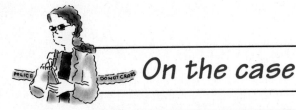

On the case

Case study background

A 56-year-old male is admitted to the medical-surgical unit with chronic obstructive pulmonary disease (COPD) and pneumonia. He has shortness of breath and audible wheezes. He's unable to answer all of the medical history questions, so his wife answers for him while he sits, leaning over the bedside table. She says he has been coughing up more sputum the past 3 days and that it's green in color. His vital signs are: oral temperature 99.2° F, pulse 115 beats/minute, respirations 28 breaths/minute and labored with accessory muscle use, and blood pressure 142/68 mm Hg. During the physical examination, the nurse notes 2+ edema of both feet and an irregular heartbeat.

His arterial blood gas results in the emergency department (ED) were pH 7.30, $Paco_2$ 65 mm Hg, Pao_2 55 mm Hg, HCO_3^- 30 mEq/L, and Sao_2 88%. The ED placed the patient on 24% oxygen by ventimask, I.V. D_5W at 50 ml/hr, methylprednisolone sodium succinate (Solu-Medrol) 40 mg I.V. q6hr, erythromycin 500 mg I.V. q6hr, breathing treatments q4hr, bed rest, and nothing-by-mouth status.

Critical thinking exercise

Complete a three-diagnosis care plan, including at least three interventions and rationales for each diagnosis, for this medical-surgical patient.

Nursing diagnosis 1

_____

Outcome

_____

Interventions	**Rationale**
1. _____	1. _____
2. _____	2. _____
3. _____	3. _____

Nursing diagnosis 2

_____

Outcome

_____

Interventions	Rationale
1. _____	1. _____
2. _____	2. _____
3. _____	3. _____

Nursing diagnosis 3

_____

Outcome

_____

Interventions	Rationale
1. _____	1. _____
2. _____	2. _____
3. _____	3. _____

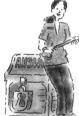

Answer key

Five potential nursing diagnoses for this patient are given in the care plan on pages 186 to 188. See how many of your diagnoses, outcomes, and interventions match. Did you think of a different diagnosis? You could be right! As long as your care plan was consistent with what you know about COPD and pneumonia, met the patient's profile, and was logically thought out, you've probably developed a good care plan.

Nursing diagnosis 1

Impaired gas exchange related to inadequate ventilation and excessive mucus production

Outcome

The patient will maintain adequate gas exchange as evidenced by return of arterial blood gas (ABG) values back to his baseline by discharge.

Intervention	Rationale
1. Assess and document respiratory rate and pattern, pulse oximetry every shift, and ABGs as ordered. Report changes.	1. Early recognition of deteriorating respiratory function can improve patient outcomes.
2. Maintain low-flow oxygen therapy as ordered.	2. Oxygen therapy helps to correct hypoxemia. High oxygen saturation levels may diminish a COPD patient's respiratory drive and cause further retention of carbon dioxide.
3. Administer bronchodilators as ordered. Watch for adverse effects of tachycardia and arrhythmias.	3. Bronchodilators relax bronchial smooth muscle, improving air flow.
4. Assist the patient to high Fowler's position as needed.	4. High Fowler's position promotes fuller lung expansion.

Nursing diagnosis 2

Ineffective airway clearance related to increased sputum production

Outcome

The patient will have a patent airway as evidenced by decreased amounts of mucus by discharge.

Interventions	Rationale
1. Assess lung sounds and respiratory rate and pattern every 4 hours and as needed.	1. Rhonchi decrease the airflow patency of large airways. Increased respiratory rate and labored breathing are signs of respiratory distress due to mucus plug or inadequate airway clearance.
2. Teach the patient effective coughing techniques.	2. Proper coughing techniques loosen mucus and ease expectoration, helping to conserve patient energy.
3. Teach the patient about adequate hydration (drinking at least six 8-ounce glasses of fluid per day, unless contraindicated).	3. Adequate hydration helps to thin secretions.
4. Perform chest physiotherapy, if ordered.	4. Chest physiotherapy helps to loosen secretions.
5. Monitor the patient's performance of incentive spirometry as ordered.	5. Incentive spirometry helps promote lung expansion.
6. Suction the patient to remove mucus from the back of the throat and mouth.	6. Thick secretions are difficult to cough out and the patient may not have the energy to do so.

Nursing diagnosis 3
Activity intolerance related to dyspnea and inadequate oxygenation

Outcome
The patient will perform activities of daily living (ADLs) with minimal assistance by discharge.

Interventions	Rationale
1. Monitor the severity of dyspnea and oxygen saturation during patient activity.	1. Activity increases oxygen demand. Assessing these variables reveals the patient's tolerance of ADLs.
2. Stop or change any activity that causes worsening dyspnea with increased heart rate.	2. Worsening dyspnea with increased heart rate signals activity intolerance, which increases the patient's oxygen demand.
3. Maintain oxygen therapy with activity as needed.	3. Oxygen helps alleviate hypoxemia and helps to improve activity tolerance.
4. Schedule activities after breathing treatments.	4. Breathing treatments maximize lung function and improve activity tolerance.
5. Help the patient to gradually increase activities every day.	5. A gradual, steady increase in activity helps to improve respiratory and cardiac condition.
6. Teach the patient to avoid factors that increase oxygen demand, such as smoking, temperature extremes, excess weight, and stress.	6. An increase in oxygen demand increases cardiac workload.
7. Teach the patient energy conservation techniques.	7. These techniques allow the patient to accomplish more with the limited energy he has.
8. Teach the patient pursed-lip and diaphragmatic breathing techniques and explain that he should use these techniques during activities.	8. These breathing techniques maximize lung function.

Nursing diagnosis 4
Risk for infection related to ineffective clearance of secretions

Outcome
The patient will verbalize methods to reduce risk of infection by discharge.

Interventions	Rationale
1. Teach the patient proper hand-washing technique.	1. Good hand washing is the single most important defense against the spread of infection.
2. Teach the patient how to care for and clean respiratory equipment at home.	2. Standing water in respiratory equipment can be a source of bacterial growth.
3. Teach the patient and family early signs of infection (increased sputum, change in sputum color, and increased dyspnea).	3. Early detection leads to early treatment and decreases the risk of complications.
4. Teach the patient about the importance of getting a yearly flu vaccine.	4. The flu vaccine provides some immunity from infection.

Nursing diagnosis 5
Anxiety related to shortness of breath

Outcome
The patient will verbalize decreased feelings of anxiety within 48 hours of admission.

Interventions	Rationale
1. Stay with the patient during episodes of shortness of breath and provide reassurance.	1. Having someone present during these episodes decreases patient anxiety.
2. Encourage the use of breathing techniques during episodes of shortness of breath and anxiety.	2. Successful use of breathing techniques helps to reduce anxiety.
3. Maintain a calm environment.	3. A calm environment promotes relaxation.
4. Teach the patient relaxation techniques, such as guided imagery and visualization.	4. Relaxation techniques help to reduce anxiety.

Part II Nursing diagnoses by medical diagnosis

8 Medical-surgical diagnoses   191

9 Maternal-neonatal diagnoses   245

10 Pediatric diagnoses   251

11 Psychiatric diagnoses   263

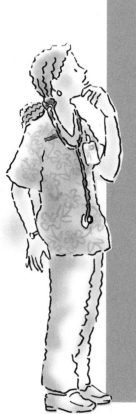

Medical-surgical diagnoses

Just the facts

In this chapter, you'll learn:

♦ nursing diagnoses that correlate with common medical-surgical medical diagnoses.

A look at medical-surgical diagnoses

This chapter covers medical-surgical problems that are common in adult patients. Each entry provides a list of a few of the major nursing diagnoses and related factors to be considered after your assessment of a patient with the particular medical diagnosis. Remember that the nursing diagnoses listed here represent the needs most commonly associated with the medical condition; your patient may have different needs.

Remember that your nursing diagnoses should be specific to the patient—not necessarily the disorder.

Abdominal aortic aneurysm repair

- Acute pain related to surgical tissue trauma
- Anxiety related to threat to health status
- Decreased cardiac output related to:
    - changes in intravascular volume
    - increased systemic vascular resistance
    - third-space fluid shift
- Deficient knowledge (preoperative and postoperative care) related to newly identified need for aortic surgery
- Ineffective breathing pattern related to:
    - effects of general anesthesia
    - endotracheal intubation
    - presence of an abdominal incision

Abdominal injury

- Acute pain related to tissue trauma
- Deficient fluid volume related to active blood loss
- Fear related to unknown diagnosis and prognosis
- Risk for infection related to:
  – penetrating wound
  – potential bowel rupture

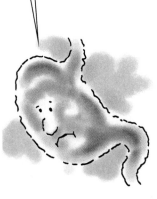

Abdominal injuries may be associated with pain or infection. Look for signs of these related problems in your patient.

Acquired immunodeficiency syndrome

- Deficient fluid volume related to persistent diarrhea associated with opportunistic infections
- Deficient knowledge (symptoms of disease progression, risk factors, transmission of disease, home care, and treatment options) related to lack of exposure to information
- Grieving related to uncertain prognosis and change in health status
- Imbalanced nutrition: Less than body requirements related to:
  – anorexia
  – diarrhea
  – medication adverse effects
  – nausea and vomiting
- Impaired gas exchange related to:
  – respiratory failure
  – ventilation-perfusion imbalance
- Impaired oral mucous membrane related to:
  – masses
  – opportunistic infections
- Impaired physical mobility related to:
  – fatigue and weakness
  – hypoxemia
  – medication adverse effects
- Ineffective airway clearance related to pneumonia
- Ineffective breathing pattern related to fatigue
- Ineffective therapeutic regimen management related to complexity of therapeutic regimen
- Risk for compromised human dignity related to societal prejudice
- Risk for impaired skin integrity related to:
  – effects of immobility
  – medication reactions
  – opportunistic disease effects
  – poor nutritional status
- Risk for infection related to immunosuppression
- Sexual dysfunction related to:
  – depression
  – fatigue
  – fear of disease transmission
  – fear of rejection

- Social isolation related to:
  - associated societal stigma
  - contacts' fear of being infected
  - fear of infection from social contacts

Acute alcohol withdrawal

- Disturbed sensory perception (visual, auditory, or tactile) related to underlying pathophysiologic changes in the nervous system
- Disturbed thought processes related to disruption in cognitive operations
- Imbalanced nutrition: Less than body requirements related to lack of food intake
- Risk for injury related to abrupt withdrawal of alcohol

Acute respiratory distress syndrome

- Deficient fluid volume related to active fluid volume loss
- Imbalanced nutrition: Less than body requirements related to inability to ingest food due to mechanical ventilation
- Impaired gas exchange related to alveolar capillary membrane changes
- Impaired skin integrity related to immobility and decreased nutritional intake
- Impaired spontaneous ventilation related to respiratory muscle fatigue
- Impaired verbal communication related to physical barriers of mechanical ventilation
- Ineffective airway clearance related to retained secretions

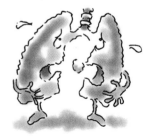

ARDS can affect everything from gas exchange and fluid volume to skin integrity and verbal communication.

Acute respiratory failure

- Activity intolerance related to respiratory distress and fatigue
- Anxiety related to sensation of severe shortness of breath
- Bathing/hygiene, dressing/grooming, toileting self care deficit related to:
  - fatigue with exertion
  - shortness of breath at rest
- Imbalanced nutrition: Less than body requirements related to shortness of breath
- Impaired gas exchange related to ventilation-perfusion imbalance
- Ineffective tissue perfusion (cardiopulmonary) related to impaired transport of oxygen across alveolar and capillary membranes

Adrenal hypofunction

- Decreased cardiac output related to altered heart rate
- Deficient fluid volume related to nausea, vomiting, and diarrhea
- Fatigue related to disease process

Alzheimer's disease

- Bathing/hygiene, dressing/grooming, feeding, toileting self-care deficit related to cognitive impairment
- Caregiver role strain related to the complexity and amount of caregiving tasks
- Chronic confusion related to degenerative loss of cerebral tissue
- Constipation related to:
  - inadequate diet
  - inadequate fluid intake
  - memory loss about toileting behavior
- Imbalanced nutrition: Less than body requirements related to:
  - difficulty swallowing
  - inadequate food intake
  - memory loss
- Impaired memory related to degenerative loss of cerebral tissue
- Risk for injury related to:
  - agnosia
  - aphasia
  - wandering behavior
- Wandering related to cognitive impairment

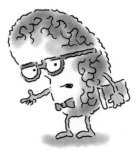

I can't remember, did you already read the nursing diagnoses that are associated with Alzheimer's disease?

Amputation

- Acute pain related to postoperative tissue, nerve, and bone trauma
- Disturbed body image related to loss of a body part
- Impaired physical mobility related to loss of a body part
- Impaired skin integrity related to traumatic or surgical tissue removal
- Risk for injury related to altered mobility

Amyotrophic lateral sclerosis

- Caregiver role strain related to complexity of care needs
- Impaired physical mobility related to muscular atrophy
- Impaired spontaneous ventilation related to respiratory muscle loss of ennervation
- Impaired swallowing related to neuromuscular impairment
- Ineffective airway clearance related to retained secretions
- Ineffective health maintenance related to lack of gross and fine motor skills

Anaphylaxis

- Death anxiety related to acute respiratory distress
- Decreased cardiac output related to altered heart rate and hypotension

• Impaired gas exchange related to edema of upper respiratory tract
• Ineffective tissue perfusion (cardiopulmonary, cerebral) related to impaired transport of oxygen across alveolar and capillary membranes

Anemia

• Activity intolerance related to weakness, fatigue, and shortness of breath
• Fatigue related to disease process
• Hopelessness related to chronic fatigue and activity intolerance
• Imbalanced nutrition: Less than body requirements related to:
  – anorexia
  – fatigue
  – lack of knowledge of need for specific nutrients (folate, iron, vitamin B_{12})
• Ineffective protection related to decreased oxygen-carrying capacity of blood
• Risk for impaired skin integrity related to:
  – decreased mobility and bed rest
  – tissue hypoxia

Aneurysm, cerebral

• Acute pain related to aneurysm
• Compromised family coping related to unknown prognosis
• Decreased intracranial adaptive capacity related to increased intracranial pressure from brain hemorrhage
• Risk for acute confusion related to moderate bleeding of cerebral artery into the brain

Aneurysm, femoral and popliteal

• Acute pain related to:
  – compression of nerves
  – edema
  – ischemia
• Deficient knowledge (preoperative and postoperative care) related to lack of exposure to information
• Ineffective tissue perfusion (peripheral) related to thrombus formation and ischemia

Aneurysm, thoracic aortic

• Acute pain related to thoracic aortic aneurysm
• Ineffective tissue perfusion (cardiopulmonary) related to aortic insufficiency
• Risk for deficient fluid volume related to compromised regulatory mechanisms

Oh no! Anaphylaxis can lead to respiratory-related death.

Aneurysm, ventricular

- Death anxiety related to risk of life-threatening rupture
- Decreased cardiac output related to arrhythmias
- Ineffective tissue perfusion (cardiopulmonary) related to heart failure

Angina pectoris

- Activity intolerance related to development of chest pain on exertion
- Anxiety related to situational crisis and shortness of breath
- Decreased cardiac output related to reduced stroke volume
- Deficient knowledge (cardiac diagnostic procedures) related to new onset of angina
- Readiness for enhanced management of therapeutic regimen related to perceived ability to reduce cardiovascular risk factors

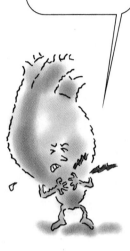

Angina pectoris can lead some patients to be intolerant of exercise.

Ankylosing spondylitis

- Activity intolerance related to pain and inflammation of joints
- Chronic pain related to deteriorating bone and cartilage of joints
- Deficient diversional activity related to pain, stiffness, and limitation of spinal motion
- Disturbed sensory perception (visual) related to eye inflammation

Appendicitis

- Acute pain related to inflammatory process
- Nausea related to peritoneal inflammation
- Risk for infection related to:
  – possible rupture of appendix
  – surgical incision

Arterial occlusive disease

- Acute pain related to arterial occlusion
- Deficient knowledge (disease and treatment options) related to lack of exposure to information
- Disturbed sensory perception (tactile) related to arterial occlusion
- Ineffective tissue perfusion (peripheral) related to reduced arterial blood flow

Atelectasis

- Anxiety related to shortness of breath
- Impaired gas exchange related to alveolar-capillary membrane changes
- Ineffective airway clearance related to excessive mucus

Basal cell epithelioma

- Disturbed body image related to cancerous lesion
- Readiness for enhanced knowledge (prevention) related to willingness to learn how to prevent recurrence
- Readiness for enhanced management of therapeutic regimen (skin care and protective measures) related to willingness to follow necessary medical regimen

Bell's palsy

- Disturbed body image related to unilateral facial weakness
- Disturbed sensory perception (gustatory) related to altered sensory reception
- Social isolation related to disturbed body image

Benign prostatic hyperplasia

- Impaired urinary elimination related to obstruction by enlarged prostate
- Risk for deficient fluid volume related to postoperative bleeding
- Sexual dysfunction related to postsurgical recovery time, retrograde ejaculation, and anxiety
- Urinary retention related to blockage by enlarged prostate

Bladder cancer

- Deficient knowledge (disease and treatment options) related to lack of exposure to information
- Fear related to unknown prognosis
- Impaired tissue integrity related to radiation or chemotherapy
- Impaired urinary elimination related to bladder irritability and pain
- Situational low self-esteem (postoperative) related to self-consciousness and disturbed self image after urinary diversion surgery

Blastomycosis

- Acute pain related to tenderness and swelling of bony lesions
- Hyperthermia related to viral infection of upper respiratory tract
- Impaired skin integrity related to macules or papules on exposed body parts
- Ineffective airway clearance related to respiratory fungal infection

Blepharitis

- Disturbed body image related to inflammation of margins of eyelids
- Effective therapeutic regimen management related to ability to manage symptoms
- Impaired skin integrity related to inflammation

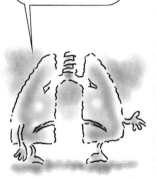

Blastomycosis originates as a respiratory infection but can end up affecting the skin and bones.

Bone tumor

- Acute pain related to pressure from tumor growth
- Anxiety related to change in health status
- Impaired physical mobility related to tumor growth or postoperative healing response
- Impaired skin integrity related to surgical incision for tumor removal

Botulism

- Death anxiety related to life-threatening disorder
- Deficient fluid volume related to vomiting and diarrhea
- Ineffective breathing pattern related to respiratory muscle failure

Brain abscess

- Acute pain related to edema and necrosis
- Ineffective tissue perfusion (cerebral) related to edema and necrosis
- Risk for acute confusion related to neurologic impairment
- Risk for injury related to neurologic impairment

Brain tumor

- Anxiety related to:
    – deterioration of physical and mental function
    – risks of treatment options
- Decreased intracranial adaptive capacity related to brain tissue injury
- Disturbed thought processes related to brain mass injury
- Impaired verbal communication related to damage to speech center
- Risk for acute confusion related to tissue damage from brain mass
- Risk for injury related to increased seizure potential and neuromuscular effects of brain tissue damage

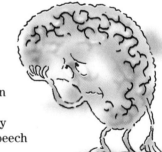

Did someone say brain tumor? Now I'm getting anxious!

Breast cancer

- Decisional conflict (treatment choice) related to risks and potential side effects of treatment options
- Disturbed body image related to breast surgery
- Fatigue related to effects of disease and treatments
- Impaired skin integrity related to incision following breast surgery
- Ineffective sexuality patterns related to perceived loss of attractiveness after mastectomy
- Stress overload related to family needs while physically and emotionally taxed

Bronchiectasis

- Imbalanced nutrition: Less than body requirements related to inadequate food intake due to illness
- Ineffective breathing pattern related to chronic abnormal dilation of bronchi and destruction of bronchial walls
- Risk for infection related to repeated damage to bronchial walls

Bronchiolitis obliterans with organizing pneumonia

- Activity intolerance related to fatigue and shortness of breath
- Imbalanced nutrition: Less than body requirements related to inadequate food intake due to disturbed taste and anorexia
- Ineffective airway clearance related to excess secretions from infection
- Ineffective breathing pattern related to inflammation of small airways

Buerger's disease

- Deficient knowledge (disease causes and risks, treatment options) related to new diagnosis
- Disturbed body image related to disease
- Ineffective tissue perfusion (peripheral) related to decreased blood flow to the feet and legs
- Risk prone health behavior related to smoking addiction

Burns

- Acute pain related to tissue destruction and exposure of nerves in partially destroyed tissue
- Compromised family coping related to prolonged disease or disability
- Contamination related to infective agents at place of injury
- Disturbed body image related to potential scarring
- Imbalanced nutrition: Less than body requirements related to increased metabolic needs of burn healing
- Impaired gas exchange related to airway burns and carbon monoxide inhalation
- Impaired physical mobility related to movement limitations from scar tissue or burn treatments
- Ineffective tissue perfusion (peripheral) related to:
  - circumferential eschar formation on arms and legs
  - compartment syndrome
  - vascular disruption
- Powerlessness related to illness
- Risk for deficient fluid volume related to active loss through disrupted skin
- Risk for imbalanced body temperature related to infection

- Risk for impaired skin integrity related to nonadherence of graft and impaired donor site healing
- Risk for infection related to:
  - decreased perfusion
  - exposure to contamination
  - impaired immunologic response
  - loss of protective integument
- Risk for injury related to continued exposure to heat or chemicals

Cancer

- Activity intolerance related to weakness from:
  - altered protein metabolism
  - cachexia
  - hypoxia
  - muscle wasting
- Anxiety related to diagnosis, treatment effects, and prognosis
- Chronic pain related to:
  - chemotherapy side effects
  - metastasis
  - primary disease
- Imbalanced nutrition: Less than body requirements related to:
  - anorexia
  - changes in taste sensation
  - stomatitis
- Impaired urinary elimination related to hemorrhagic cystitis from chemotherapy
- Ineffective sexuality patterns related to alterations in body image
- Readiness for enhanced hope related to decreased signs of cancer on repeated testing and healthful changes in lifestyle to decrease risk of recurrence
- Risk for constipation related to opioid use
- Risk for infection related to immunosuppression from chemotherapy and malnutrition
- Risk for peripheral neurovascular dysfunction related to peripheral neuropathies caused by chemotherapy
- Risk for situational low self-esteem related to:
  - hair loss
  - role changes
  - weight loss
- Sleep deprivation related to:
  - alterations in patterns of elimination
  - anxiety
  - fear of dying while sleeping
  - other sequelae of cancer
  - pain

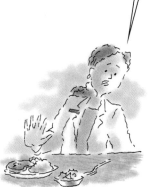

Patients with cancer can experience imbalanced nutrition as a result of anorexia, changes in taste, and stomatitis. Nothing for me right now, thanks.

Candidiasis

- Impaired oral mucous membrane related to fungal infection in mouth
- Impaired skin integrity related to fungal infection
- Ineffective thermoregulation related to systemic infection
- Risk for impaired liver function related to fluconazole (Diflucan) or other specific systemic antifungal agents

Cardiac arrhythmias

- Activity intolerance related to shortness of breath or chest pain when dysrhythmic or drug effects
- Anxiety related to change in health status
- Decreased cardiac output related to altered contractility of heart muscle
- Deficient knowledge (disease and treatment options) related to lack of exposure to information
- Fatigue related to arrhythmias
- Fear related to decreased confidence in health status
- Ineffective coping related to inadequate level of control over illness recurrence
- Ineffective tissue perfusion (cardiopulmonary) related to impaired cardiac cycle and blood oxygenation

Cardiac surgery

- Acute confusion related to:
  - anesthesia
  - cerebral ischemia or infarction
  - sensory overload from intensive care unit environment
- Deficient fluid volume related to blood loss
- Deficient knowledge (postoperative care) related to complex therapeutic regimen
- Dysfunctional ventilatory weaning response related to respiratory complications postoperatively
- Impaired gas exchange related to:
  - alveolar collapse
  - increased pulmonary shunt
  - increased secretions
  - pain

Cardiac tamponade

- Decreased cardiac output related to altered preload
- Fear related to life-threatening disorder
- Ineffective breathing pattern related to cardiac tamponade

Cardiogenic shock

- Activity intolerance related to:
  - diminished cardiovascular reserve
  - hypoxemia
  - weakness
- Decreased cardiac output related to heart rate abnormalities or diminished contractility
- Excess fluid volume related to compromised regulatory mechanisms
- Impaired gas exchange related to ventilation-perfusion imbalance

Cardiomyopathy

- Anxiety related to deterioration in health status (medication effects and adverse effects)
- Decreased cardiac output related to arrhythmias and ineffective pump function
- Deficient knowledge (disease and treatment) related to changes in regimen
- Ineffective breathing pattern related to disease process

Carotid endarterectomy

- Anxiety related to threat to health status
- Deficient knowledge (procedure) related to unfamiliarity with procedure and hospital protocol
- Impaired gas exchange related to airway obstruction from tracheal compression or aspiration
- Risk for infection related to surgical incision

Carpal tunnel syndrome

- Acute pain related to nerve compression
- Bathing or hygiene self-care deficit related to pain
- Risk for peripheral neurovascular dysfunction related to disease process

Cataract

- Deficient knowledge (disease and treatment options) related to lack of exposure to information
- Disturbed sensory perception (visual) related to cataract
- Impaired physical mobility related to fear of injury
- Risk for injury related to impaired vision

Cerebral contusion

- Acute pain related to headache after trauma
- Disturbed sensory perception (auditory, olfactory, visual) related to bruising of brain tissue

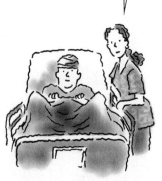

Disturbances in auditory, olfactory, and visual perception can result from cerebral contusion.

- Risk for acute confusion related to brain injury
- Risk for injury related to brain injury

Cervical cancer

- Acute pain related to tumor invasion
- Deficient knowledge (disease and treatment options) related to lack of exposure to information
- Disturbed body image related to weight loss
- Fatigue related to cancer process and treatment effects
- Sexual dysfunction related to postcoital pain and bleeding

Chest injury, blunt

- Acute pain related to injury
- Anxiety related to impaired oxygenation
- Impaired spontaneous ventilation related to blunt trauma
- Ineffective breathing pattern related to chest wall injury

Chlamydia

- Deficient knowledge (disease and treatment options) related to lack of information on sexually transmitted diseases
- Ineffective sexuality patterns related to fear of spreading infection
- Risk for infection related to untreated partners

Cholecystectomy

- Acute pain related to gallbladder inflammation
- Imbalanced nutrition: Less than body requirements related to:
  - altered lipid metabolism
  - increased nutritional needs during healing
  - nasogastric (NG) suction
  - postoperative nothing-by-mouth (NPO) status
  - preoperative nausea and vomiting
- Impaired oral mucous membrane related to NPO status and possible NG suction
- Ineffective breathing pattern related to pain from high abdominal incision
- Risk for infection (postoperative) related to obstruction of external biliary drainage tube

Cholelithiasis, cholecystitis

- Acute pain related to gallbladder inflammation or presence of stones
- Imbalanced nutrition: Less than body requirements related to attacks following meals
- Risk for infection related to complications of disease

Chronic alcoholism

- Dysfunctional family processes: Alcoholism related to alcohol abuse
- Imbalanced nutrition: Less than body requirements related to lack of food intake
- Ineffective coping related to:
  – anger
  – denial
  – dependence
- Ineffective therapeutic regimen management related to denial of problem
- Risk for impaired liver function related to alcohol intake
- Risk for other-directed violence related to:
  – disorientation
  – impaired judgment
- Risk prone health behavior related to alcohol abuse

Chronic fatigue and immune dysfunction syndrome

- Fatigue related to illness
- Hopelessness related to chronic illness
- Sleep deprivation related to internal factors

Chronic obstructive pulmony disease

- Activity intolerance related to shortness of breath
- Adult failure to thrive related to fatigue and chronic dyspnea of severe disease
- Deficient knowledge (disease processes and treatment) related to complexity of disorder
- Imbalanced nutrition: Less than body requirements related to shortness of breath during and after meals
- Impaired gas exchange related to impaired excretion of carbon dioxide
- Impaired home maintenance related to inadequate support systems and inability to do tasks due to disease process
- Ineffective breathing pattern related to fatigue, or blunting of respiratory drive
- Ineffective sexuality patterns related to:
  – adverse reactions to medications
  – change in body image
  – change in relationship with spouse or partner
  – deconditioning
  – shortness of breath
- Insomnia related to:
  – anxiety
  – bronchodilator's stimulant effect
  – depression
  – shortness of breath

Cirrhosis

- Dysfunctional family processes: Alcoholism related to alcohol addiction
- Excess fluid volume related to fluid retention
- Imbalanced nutrition: Less than body requirements related to:
  - GI symptoms (anorexia, nausea, vomiting, diarrhea)
  - inability to absorb nutrients
- Impaired gas exchange related to ventilation-perfusion imbalance
- Risk for acute confusion related to increasing ammonia levels
- Risk for impaired liver function related to alcohol addiction
- Risk for impaired skin integrity related to edema and pruritus

Clostridium difficile infection

- Anxiety related to change in health status
- Risk for deficient fluid volume related to diarrhea
- Risk for impaired skin integrity related to diarrhea
- Risk for infection related to inadequate defenses

Cold injury

- Deficient knowledge (prevention of cold injury) related to inexperience with excessive cold
- Hypothermia related to cold injury
- Risk for impaired skin integrity related to frostbite

Colorectal cancer

- Constipation related to GI obstruction
- Diarrhea related to inflammation or malabsorption
- Fatigue related to malnutrition or anemia
- Imbalanced nutrition: Less than body requirements related to inability to absorb nutrients
- Risk for deficient fluid volume related to diarrhea or bleeding
- Risk for spiritual distress related to potential life-threatening diagnosis

Colostomy

- Deficient knowledge (care of descending or sigmoid colostomy) related to unfamiliarity with altered bowel procedures
- Disturbed body image related to loss of control over fecal elimination
- Risk for impaired skin integrity related to fecal contamination of skin
- Sexual dysfunction related to change in body image

Concussion

- Disturbed sensory perception (visual) related to a blow to the head
- Nausea related to blow to the head
- Risk for injury related to dizziness and lethargy

Conjunctivitis

- Risk for impaired skin integrity related to eye discharge and tearing
- Risk for infection related to contagious disease and ability to spread to other eye or other people
- Risk for situational low self-esteem related to hyperemia of eyes

Cor pulmonale

- Activity intolerance related to exertional dyspnea
- Decreased cardiac output related to decreased stroke volume
- Grieving related to poor prognosis
- Impaired gas exchange related to pulmonary capillary destruction

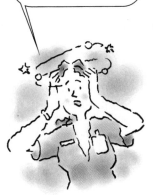

A patient with a concussion is at risk for injuries related to dizziness and lethargy. Now that's a blow to the head!

Corneal abrasion

- Acute pain related to eye injury
- Disturbed sensory perception (visual) related to eye injury
- Risk for injury related to poor visual acuity

Corneal ulcer

- Disturbed sensory perception (visual) related to corneal ulcer
- Risk for infection related to inadequate primary defenses
- Risk for injury related to visual blurring

Coronary artery disease

- Anxiety related to angina
- Decreased cardiac output related to diminished coronary blood flow
- Health-seeking behaviors (learning about risk factors) related to perceived ability to decrease risk factors
- Ineffective family therapeutic regimen management related to disinterest in learning emergency care procedures (use of nitroglycerin, when to call 911, cardiopulmonary resuscitation)
- Ineffective tissue perfusion (cardiopulmonary) related to atherosclerosis

Craniotomy

- Deficient knowledge (impending craniotomy) related to lack of exposure to information
- Disturbed body image related to hair loss and possible disruption of motor function
- Risk for deficient fluid volume related to:

    – diuretic therapy
    – fluid restriction
    – GI suction
    – hyperthermia
- Risk for infection related to invasive techniques (surgery, continuous intracranial monitoring, ventricular drains)
- Risk for injury related to:
    – decreased level of consciousness
    – drug therapy
    – effect of anesthetics
    – seizures

Crohn's disease (irritable bowel syndrome)

- Acute pain related to bowel inflammation
- Compromised family coping related to chronic disease
- Diarrhea related to bowel inflammation
- Nausea related to bowel inflammation
- Risk for imbalanced fluid volume related to diarrhea
- Risk for infection related to invasive procedures (surgery, home infusions)

Cushing's syndrome

- Disturbed body image related to secondary effects of excessive corticosteroid levels
- Excess fluid volume related to high serum corticosteroid levels
- Risk for impaired skin integrity related to secondary effects of medications
- Risk for infection related to the immunosuppressive action of glucocorticoids
- Risk for unstable glucose level related to the anti-insulin properties of glucocorticoids

Dermatitis

- Chronic low self-esteem related to poor body image
- Impaired skin integrity related to inflammation, itching, or lesions of the skin
- Risk for infection related to inadequate primary defenses

Dermatophytosis

- Acute pain related to inflammation
- Impaired skin integrity related to skin infection
- Readiness for enhanced management of therapeutic regimen related to desire to follow through with treatment regimen

Diabetes insipidus

- Constipation related to dehydration
- Deficient fluid volume related to active fluid loss
- Impaired oral mucous membrane related to dehydration

> Watch for signs of dehydration in a patient with diabetes insipidus. Fluid volume can be difficult to balance.

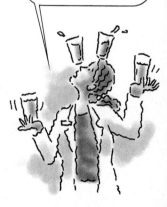

Diabetes mellitus

- Compromised family coping related to prolonged disease
- Deficient knowledge (self-care) related to complex chronic disease
- Ineffective therapeutic regimen management related to:
  - ineffective coping with chronic disorders
  - lack of material resources
  - lack of support
- Ineffective tissue perfusion (renal, peripheral) related to complications of disease
- Risk for imbalanced nutrition: More than body requirements related to excessive calorie intake
- Risk for unstable glucose level related to:
  - inadequate endogenous insulin (type 1)
  - inadequate endogenous insulin and insulin resistance (type 2)

Diabetic ketoacidosis

- Deficient fluid volume related to osmotic diuresis or vomiting
- Deficient knowledge (self-care) related to lack of exposure to complex disease and therapy information
- Risk for injury related to:
  - acidosis
  - cerebral dehydration
  - decreased perfusion
  - hypoxemia
- Risk for unstable glucose level related to decreased cellular glucose uptake and use

Dislocation and subluxation

- Acute pain related to damage to tissue
- Anxiety related to pain and treatment
- Impaired physical mobility related to joint injury and pain

Disseminated intravascular coagulation

- Acute pain related to:
  - bleeding into organ or joint capsules
  - hematomas
  - tissue ischemia
- Deficient fluid volume related to hemorrhage
- Fear related to unfamiliarity with hospital environment
- Impaired gas exchange related to hypoxemia
- Impaired skin integrity related to capillary fragility

Diverticulitis

- Acute pain related to:
  - bowel infection or perforation
  - inflammation

- Constipation related to lack of roughage in diet
- Deficient fluid volume related to active loss and poor intake
- Diarrhea related to inflammation and infection

Drug overdose

- Hopelessness related to:
  - emotional disorganization
  - inadequate resources
  - low self-esteem
- Ineffective airway clearance related to:
  - decreased or absent gag reflex
  - lavage procedures
  - obstruction by tongue
  - reduced alertness
  - vomiting
- Risk prone health behavior related to drug addiction

Duodenal ulcer

- Chronic pain related to:
  - excessive motility of upper GI tract
  - increased hydrochloric acid secretion
  - increased spasm
  - inflammation of the duodenum
  - intragastric pressure
- Imbalanced nutrition: Less than body requirements related to:
  - dysphagia
  - mouth soreness
  - nausea and vomiting
- Risk for deficient fluid volume related to:
  - diarrhea
  - GI hemorrhage
  - vomiting

Ebola virus infection

- Diarrhea related to viral infection
- Fear related to poor prognosis
- Grieving related to probable death from disease
- Hyperthermia related to infection
- Impaired skin integrity related to diarrhea
- Risk for deficient fluid volume related to diarrhea and hemorrhage

Encephalitis

- Acute pain related to increased intracranial pressure
- Disturbed thought processes related to cerebral edema
- Hyperthermia related to infection
- Impaired physical mobility related to possible coma

Endocarditis
- Activity intolerance related to fatigue and weakness
- Decreased cardiac output related to bacterial or fungal invasion of heart
- Hyperthermia related to infection

Endometriosis
- Acute pain related to inflammation and adhesions of endometrial tissue
- Deficient knowledge (disease and treatment options) related to lack of exposure to information
- Sexual dysfunction related to pain

Epididymitis
- Acute pain related to infection
- Risk for infection related to inadequate primary defenses
- Sexual dysfunction related to pain, swelling, and tenderness of groin area

Epilepsy
- Deficient knowledge (disease) related to lack of exposure to information
- Fatigue related to antiseizure medication side effect
- Readiness for enhanced management of therapeutic regimen related to readiness to follow treatment
- Risk for caregiver role strain related to worry and fear about diagnosis
- Risk for compromised human dignity related to seizures

Escherichia coli and other Enterobacteriaceae infections
- Acute pain related to crampy diarrhea
- Deficient fluid volume related to loss through diarrhea and vomiting
- Diarrhea related to infection

Esophageal cancer
- Acute pain related to:
  - fistula
  - surgery
  - tumor
- Fatigue related to cachexia
- Imbalanced nutrition: Less than body requirements related to dysphasia
- Risk for aspiration related to dysphasia

Esophageal diverticula

- Imbalanced nutrition: Less than body requirements related to dysphasia and regurgitation
- Risk for aspiration related to dysphasia and regurgitation
- Risk for infection related to inadequate primary defenses

Extraocular motor nerve palsy

- Anxiety related to chronic disease
- Bathing/hygiene or feeding self-care deficit related to vision impairment
- Deficient diversional activity related to vision impairment
- Disturbed sensory perception (visual) related to dysfunction of cranial nerves

Fatty liver

- Acute pain related to large, tender liver
- Deficient knowledge (proper diet) related to lack of exposure to information
- Imbalanced nutrition: Less than body requirements related to anorexia and liver inflammation
- Imbalanced nutrition: More than body requirements related to excess fat and calorie consumption
- Risk for impaired liver function related to excess fat accumulation in the liver

Femoral popliteal bypass

- Acute pain related to surgical incision
- Impaired physical mobility related to surgery and preexisting disability
- Impaired skin integrity related to surgical incision and preexisting stasis ulcers
- Ineffective tissue perfusion (peripheral) related to arterial insufficiency
- Risk for infection related to inadequate primary defenses (broken skin)

Fibromyalgia syndrome

- Chronic pain related to illness
- Fatigue related to musculoskeletal pain and sleep disturbance
- Insomnia related to pain

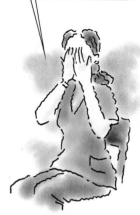

Patients with extraocular motor nerve palsy may be limited in the activities in which they can participate. I can see why. I mean, I can't see why?!

Gastric cancer

- Deficient fluid volume related to vomiting and decreased fluid intake
- Delayed surgical recovery related to decreased nutrition and primary defenses
- Imbalanced nutrition: Less than body requirements related to:
  - a feeling of fullness after eating
  - dyspepsia
  - epigastric discomfort
- Risk for spiritual distress related to cancer diagnosis and prognosis

Gastritis

- Acute pain related to inflammation
- Deficient knowledge (prevention and treatment) related to lack of exposure to smoking, diet information, and medication use
- Nausea related to gastric irritation
- Readiness for enhanced nutrition related to willingness to ingest nonirritating foods

Gastroenteritis

- Acute pain related to intestinal flu
- Nausea related to bacteria, parasites, and virus in intestine
- Risk for deficient fluid volume related to nausea and vomiting
- Risk for imbalanced body temperature related to infection

Gastroesophageal reflux

- Chronic pain related to reflux of gastric and duodenal contents into esophagus
- Deficient knowledge (treatment options) related to lack of exposure to information
- Risk for aspiration related to reflux

Gastrointestinal hemorrhage

- Deficient fluid volume related to active bleeding
- Deficient knowledge (potential recurrent bleeding) related to unfamiliarity with disorder
- Fear related to sight of blood and distressing physical symptoms
- Risk for injury related to:
  - accumulation of toxins
  - electrolyte imbalance
  - inadequate organ perfusion
  - ulcer perforation
  - undetected bleeding

Glaucoma

- Anxiety related to progression of disease
- Deficient knowledge (eyedrops administration procedures) related to lack of previous experience
- Disturbed sensory perception (visual) related to high intraocular pressure and damage to optic nerve
- Risk for injury related to loss of peripheral vision

Glomerulonephritis

- Excess fluid volume related to oliguria
- Imbalanced nutrition: Less than body requirements related to anorexia
- Ineffective tissue perfusion (renal) related to disease process
- Risk for infection related to inadequate defenses

Goiter

- Disturbed body image related to neck distention
- Impaired swallowing related to swelling and distention of neck
- Ineffective breathing pattern related to compression of trachea

Gonorrhea

- Ineffective sexuality patterns related to fear of spreading infection
- Risk for infection related to inadequate primary resources
- Risk for situational low self-esteem related to infection

Gout

- Activity intolerance related to painful joints
- Acute pain related to urate deposits in joints
- Disturbed body image related to joint deformity

Graft rejection syndrome

- Grieving related to loss of graft
- Ineffective tissue perfusion (peripheral, cardiopulmonary, renal) related to stimulation of the complement cascade with resultant thrombosis and tissue infarction
- Powerlessness related to loss of graft

Granulocytopenia, lymphocytopenia

- Deficient knowledge (disease and treatment options) related to lack of exposure to information
- Fatigue related to low white blood cell (WBC) count
- Hyperthermia related to infection
- Risk for infection related to low WBC count

Guillain-Barré syndrome

- Bathing/hygiene, feeding, toileting self-care deficit related to muscle weakness and paralysis
- Fear related to sudden onset of illness
- Impaired spontaneous ventilation related to muscle weakness and paralysis
- Ineffective airway clearance related to neuromuscular dysfunction
- Risk for urge urinary incontinence related to muscle weakness

Hantavirus pulmonary syndrome

- Hyperthermia related to infection
- Impaired gas exchange related to respiratory failure and ventilation-perfusion imbalance
- Ineffective breathing pattern related to pulmonary infiltrates with respiratory compromise

Headache

- Acute pain related to vascular, muscle contraction
- Fatigue related to headache
- Ineffective coping related to recurrence of headaches

Hearing loss

- Disturbed sensory perception (auditory) related to hearing loss
- Readiness for enhanced communication related to ability to learn ways to communicate without adequate hearing
- Risk for injury related to not hearing danger signs in environment

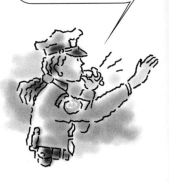

Your patient's hearing loss can affect his ability to hear danger signals in the environment, putting him at risk for injury.

Heart failure

- Decreased cardiac output related to:
  – altered heart rhythm
  – decreased contractility
  – fluid volume overload
  – increased afterload
- Deficient knowledge (treatment regimen) related to lack of exposure to information
- Excess fluid volume related to:
  – decreased myocardial contractility
  – decreased renal perfusion
  – increased sodium and water retention
- Imbalanced nutrition: Less than body requirements related to decreased appetite and unpalatability of low-sodium diet
- Ineffective breathing pattern related to fatigue
- Ineffective therapeutic regimen management related to:
  – complexity of regimen
  – health beliefs
  – negative relationship with caregivers
- Powerlessness related to illness

Heat syndrome

- Deficient knowledge (management of syndrome) related to lack of exposure to information
- Deficient knowledge (prevention of heat syndrome) related to language barrier or impaired literacy, or lack of exposure to information
- Hyperthermia related to environmental heat conditions

Hemophilia

- Anxiety related to risk of acute bleeding
- Ineffective protection related to abnormal blood profile
- Risk for injury related to lack of awareness of environmental dangers
- Risk for trauma related to external factors

Hemorrhoids

- Acute pain related to inflammation of hemorrhoid veins
- Constipation related to pain
- Deficient knowledge (activities that increase intravenous pressure) related to lack of exposure to information

Hemothorax

- Acute pain related to blood in pleural cavity
- Anxiety related to acute shortness of breath
- Fear related to sudden onset of injury
- Ineffective breathing pattern related to blood in pleural cavity

Hepatic encephalopathy

- Deficient fluid volume related to active loss
- Disturbed thought processes related to ammonia intoxication of the brain
- Risk for impaired liver function related to alcohol abuse

Hepatitis

- Acute pain related to inflammation of the liver
- Deficient knowledge (home care, disease process, prevention of recurrence) related to lack of exposure to information
- Fatigue related to disease process
- Imbalanced nutrition: Less than body requirements related to anorexia, diarrhea, nausea, or vomiting
- Nausea related to GI irritation
- Risk for activity intolerance related to increased fatigue
- Risk for deficient fluid volume related to vomiting and diarrhea
- Risk for impaired skin integrity related to:
  - frequent diarrhea
  - prolonged bed rest
  - pruritus

Herniated disk

- Activity intolerance related to pain
- Acute pain related to impingement on spinal nerve roots
- Readiness for enhanced management of therapeutic regimen related to ability to follow through with regimen

Herpes simplex

- Acute pain related to cold sores and fever blisters
- Chronic low self-esteem related to skin lesions
- Ineffective sexuality patterns related to fear of spreading infection to sexual partner
- Sexual dysfunction related to sexually transmitted disease (herpes simplex 2)

Herpes zoster

- Acute pain related to inflammation of the dorsal root ganglia
- Chronic pain related to postherpetic neuralgia
- Hyperthermia related to infection
- Impaired skin integrity related to localized vesicular skin lesions

Hiatal hernia

- Acute pain related to displacement or stretching of the stomach
- Deficient knowledge (treatment options) related to lack of exposure to information
- Impaired swallowing related to esophagitis, ulcers, or strictures

Hodgkin's disease

- Fatigue related to weight loss and disease process
- Grieving related to perceived potential for loss of life
- Hyperthermia related to immunosuppression
- Ineffective protection related to Hodgkin's disease

Huntington's disease

- Bathing/hygiene, dressing/grooming, feeding, toileting self-care deficit related to physical deterioration
- Bowel incontinence related to neuromuscular impairment
- Caregiver role strain related to complexity and amount of caregiving activities
- Disturbed thought processes related to brain involvement
- Impaired physical mobility related to neuromuscular impairment
- Impaired verbal communication related to dysarthria

Hydronephrosis

- Acute pain related to physical obstruction of urine flow
- Impaired urinary elimination related to obstruction of urine flow
- Risk for infection related to obstruction of urine flow

Hyperaldosteronism

- Deficient knowledge (disease) related to lack of exposure to information
- Fatigue related to hypokalemia
- Impaired urinary elimination related to polyuria and polydipsia
- Risk for unstable glucose level related to hypokalemia

Hyperparathyroidism

- Acute pain related to hypercalcemia, which causes bone tenderness, pancreatitis, and peptic ulcers
- Hopelessness related to deteriorating condition
- Imbalanced nutrition: Less than body requirements related to nausea and vomiting

Hyperosmolar hyperglycemic nonketotic syndrome

- Deficient fluid volume related to osmotic diuresis
- Deficient knowledge (self-care) related to lack of exposure to complex disease and management
- Risk for injury related to:
  - cerebral dehydration
  - cerebral edema during rapid rehydration
  - decreased perfusion
  - glucose deprivation
  - hypoxemia
- Risk for unstable glucose level related to inadequate insulin secretion or peripheral insulin resistance

Hypertension

- Decreased cardiac output related to decreased stroke volume
- Excess fluid volume related to compromised regulatory mechanisms
- Ineffective therapeutic regimen management related to deficient knowledge
- Noncompliance (treatment) related to health beliefs and cultural influences

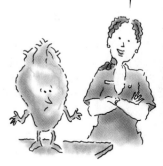

Patients with hypertension can be noncompliant as a result of health beliefs or cultural influences.

Hypoglycemia

- Fatigue related to hypoglycemia
- Ineffective therapeutic regimen management related to complexity of the disease and deficient knowledge
- Risk for injury related to:
  - excessive exercise
  - inappropriate exogenous insulin use
  - lack of food

Hypoparathyroidism

- Decreased cardiac output related to cardiac arrhythmias
- Imbalanced nutrition: Less than body requirements related to inability to ingest foods due to dysphagia
- Ineffective coping related to situational crisis

Hypothyroidism

- Decreased cardiac output related to cardiac arrhythmias
- Disturbed body image related to periorbital edema and upper eyelid droop
- Disturbed thought processes related to decreasing mental stability and forgetfulness
- Risk for imbalanced body temperature related to decreased sensitivity of thermoreceptors

Hypovolemic shock

- Decreased cardiac output related to altered heart rate and rhythm
- Impaired gas exchange related to ventilation-perfusion imbalance
- Ineffective coping related to threat to life
- Ineffective tissue perfusion (cerebral, cardiopulmonary, renal, peripheral) related to hypovolemia
- Risk for deficient fluid volume related to:
  - disease processes
  - iatrogenic interventions
  - surgical interventions
- Risk for injury related to complications from ischemia

Ileal conduit urinary diversion

- Deficient knowledge (care of an ileal conduit) related to lack of exposure to information
- Disturbed body image related to urinary diversion
- Impaired urinary elimination related to creation of an ileal conduit
- Risk for infection related to GI or genitourinary anastomosis breakdown or leakage
- Sexual dysfunction related to cystectomy and possible ejaculatory incompetence with prostatectomy

Infertility

- Complicated grieving related to multiple miscarriages
- Ineffective coping related to uncertainty of future pregnancies
- Situational low self-esteem related to infertility

Inflammatory bowel disease

- Chronic pain related to abdominal distention
- Deficient fluid volume related to decreased fluid intake and increased fluid loss through diarrhea

- Imbalanced nutrition: Less than body requirements related to:
  - decreased nutrient intake
  - increased nutrient loss
  - possible decreased bowel absorption
- Impaired skin integrity related to frequent stools and altered nutritional status
- Ineffective sexuality patterns related to diminished physical energy and persistence of uncomfortable physical symptoms
- Insomnia related to:
  - anxiety related to hospitalization
  - nocturnal defecation
  - uncomfortable sensations
- Risk for infection related to:
  - bowel perforation
  - general debilitation
  - immunosuppression
- Social isolation related to dependent behavior

Influenza

- Hyperthermia related to infection
- Ineffective community therapeutic regimen management related to insufficient supply of influenza vaccine
- Risk for imbalanced fluid volume related to fever, cough, decreased oral intake
- Risk for infection related to inadequate primary and secondary defenses to prevent secondary bacterial invasion

Inguinal hernia

- Acute pain related to tension on herniated contents
- Ineffective tissue perfusion (gastrointestinal) related to diversion of bowel through hernia
- Risk for infection related to complete obstruction

Intestinal obstruction

- Acute pain related to abdominal distention
- Constipation related to intestinal obstruction
- Ineffective tissue perfusion (gastrointestinal) related to obstruction
- Risk for deficient fluid volume related to intestinal obstruction

Joint replacement

- Acute pain related to surgery
- Impaired physical mobility related to joint surgery
- Risk for infection related to incision

Kaposi's sarcoma

- Acute pain related to lesions that break down or impinge on nerves and organs
- Grieving related to threat of death in advanced disease and when associated with human immunodeficiency virus
- Impaired skin integrity related to disease process
- Ineffective breathing pattern related to bronchial blockage and hypoventilation

Kidney transplant

- Acute pain related to frequent invasive procedures and surgery
- Disturbed body image related to effects of steroid therapy
- Excess fluid volume related to function of transplanted kidney
- Ineffective coping related to sensory overload
- Noncompliance (drug regimen) related to adverse drug effects and complicated multidrug regimen
- Risk for infection related to immunosuppression

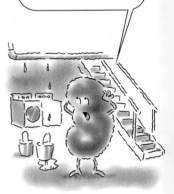

Your patient may have excess fluid volume related to the function of his transplanted kidney. My pail runneth over...

Laminectomy

- Acute pain related to:
  - immobility
  - muscle spasm
  - paresthesia secondary to surgical trauma and postoperative edema
- Deficient knowledge (preoperative and postoperative care) related to lack of exposure to information
- Ineffective tissue perfusion (renal) related to:
  - anesthesia
  - anxiety
  - cord edema
  - injury to the spinal nerve roots innervating the bladder
  - opioids
  - pain
  - supine positioning
- Risk for deficient fluid volume related to:
  - blood loss during surgery
  - hemorrhage at the incision site
  - retroperitoneal hemorrhage
  - vascular injury

Laryngeal cancer

- Acute pain related to drinking citrus or hot liquid or tumor pressure
- Grieving related to potential loss of significant other
- Imbalanced nutrition: Less than body requirements related to impaired swallowing
- Impaired swallowing related to tumor
- Impaired verbal communication related to laryngectomy

Legionnaires' disease

- Diarrhea related to infection
- Fatigue related to infection
- Hyperthermia related to infection
- Ineffective airway clearance related to increased mucus production
- Risk for infection related to inadequate immune defenses to prevent secondary bacterial invasion

Leukemia

- Activity intolerance related to:
  – depressed nutritional status
  – fatigue secondary to rapid destruction of leukemic cells
  – tissue hypoxia secondary to anemia
- Acute pain related to physical, biological, or chemical agents
- Deficient knowledge (therapeutic modality and choice and care of vascular access device) related to lack of exposure to information
- Fatigue related to rapid destruction of leukemic cells
- Hopelessness related to prognosis
- Imbalanced nutrition: Less than body requirements related to:
  – anorexia
  – chemotherapy
  – nausea
  – taste perception changes
  – vomiting
- Impaired oral mucous membrane related to:
  – cytotoxic effects of chemotherapy
  – immunosuppression secondary to disease
- Ineffective coping related to uncertain prognosis and multiple disease- and treatment-induced losses
- Ineffective protection related to severe immunosuppression associated with bone marrow transplantation or peripheral stem cell transplantation protocol
- Readiness for enhanced immunization status related to successful bone marrow transplantation
- Risk for deficient fluid volume related to risk of hemorrhage
- Risk for infection related to immunosuppression

Liver abscess

- Acute pain related to liver abscess
- Anxiety related to change in health status
- Impaired gas exchange related to abnormal breathing rate and rhythm due to pain
- Risk for imbalanced body temperature related to infection

Liver failure

- Imbalanced nutrition: Less than body requirements related to catabolism caused by liver disease
- Impaired skin integrity related to:
  - ascites
  - increased bleeding tendencies
  - jaundice
  - malnutrition
- Risk for acute confusion related to hepatic encephalopathy syndrome
- Risk for imbalanced fluid volume related to ascites
- Risk for infection related to liver disease

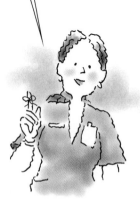

Remember that every patient may have different needs. The nursing diagnoses listed here are those that are most commonly associated with each medical condition.

Liver transplantation

- Acute pain related to surgery
- Compromised family coping related to prolonged disease
- Imbalanced nutrition: Less than body requirements related to:
  - anorexia
  - chronic illness
  - initial postoperative nothing-by-mouth status
- Ineffective breathing pattern related to prolonged general anesthesia and a large abdominal incision
- Readiness for enhanced hope related to new liver
- Risk for deficient fluid volume related to high-dose steroid therapy and fluid loss
- Risk for impaired liver function related to surgery and disease process
- Risk for infection related to surgical incision and immunosuppression

Lung abscess

- Hyperthermia related to infection
- Impaired gas exchange related to altered oxygen supply
- Ineffective airway clearance related to increased secretions

Lung cancer

- Activity intolerance related to imbalance between oxygen supply and demand
- Imbalanced nutrition: Less than body requirements related to inability to ingest food
- Ineffective airway clearance related to fatigue
- Powerlessness related to perceived mortality

Lupus erythematosus

- Decreased cardiac output related to pericarditis, myocarditis, or endocarditis
- Hyperthermia related to immunosuppression
- Impaired physical mobility related to joint inflammation
- Impaired skin integrity related to rashes
- Risk prone health behavior related to disability

Lyme disease

- Acute pain related to arthritis
- Anxiety related to long treatment course
- Fatigue related to infection
- Impaired skin integrity related to rash

Lymphoma, non-Hodgkin's

- Anxiety related to unknown hospital procedures and threat to health status
- Deficient knowledge (self-care of vascular access device, including peripherally or centrally inserted venous catheters or subcutaneous ports) related to lack of exposure to information
- Disturbed body image related to effects of chemotherapy or radiation therapy
- Imbalanced nutrition: Less than body requirements related to:
  - altered oral mucous membrane
  - anorexia
  - fatigue
  - nausea and vomiting
  - taste alterations
- Impaired skin integrity related to effects of radiation therapy
- Ineffective protection related to immunosuppression
- Risk for infection related to:
  - chemotherapy
  - leukopenia, lymphopenia from bone marrow involvement
  - radiation therapy effects

Macular degeneration

- Disturbed sensory perception (visual) related to aging process
- Impaired physical mobility related to vision impairment
- Powerlessness related to illness progression

Malignant melanoma

- Disturbed body image related to skin lesion on head or neck
- Impaired skin integrity related to sore, inflamed, itchy skin lesion
- Readiness for enhanced management of therapeutic regimen related to understanding treatment protocols

Mastectomy

- Anxiety related to fear of cancer recurrence
- Deficient knowledge (treatment options) related to lack of exposure to information
- Disturbed body image related to loss of a body part
- Risk for infection related to incision

Mechanical ventilation

- Bathing/hygiene, dressing/grooming, feeding, toileting self-care deficit related to impaired mobility status, pain
- Deficient fluid volume related to:
  - altered oral intake
  - fluid retention
  - osmotic diuresis
- Deficient knowledge (peripheral parenteral nutrition [PPN] catheter care and therapy) related to lack of experience with PPN
- Fear related to inability to speak and dependence on life support
- Imbalanced nutrition: Less than body requirements related to inability to ingest nutrients orally or digest them satisfactorily, or to increased need
- Impaired bed mobility related to ventilator
- Impaired gas exchange related to insufficient oxygen levels
- Ineffective airway clearance related to:
  - increased secretions
  - presence of an endotracheal tube
  - underlying disease
- Risk for impaired skin integrity related to physical immobility
- Risk for infection related to central venous catheter
- Risk for injury related to complications of PPN catheter insertion

- Risk for injury related to:
  - bypassed safety alarm mechanisms
  - increased intrathoracic pressure
  - mechanical breakdown
  - patient deterioration

Ménière's disease

- Deficient knowledge (symptom prevention and control measures) related to recent onset of disease
- Disturbed sensory perception (auditory, kinesthetic) related to disease process
- Impaired physical mobility related to vertigo

Meningitis

- Acute pain related to headache, joint involvement, muscle aches from infection
- Hyperthermia related to infection
- Ineffective tissue perfusion (cerebral) related to increased intracranial pressure
- Risk for injury related to seizures

Metabolic acidosis

- Acute confusion related to increased body acid
- Deficient fluid volume related to active loss from diarrhea and vomiting
- Ineffective breathing pattern related to fatigue and Kussmaul's respirations
- Nausea related to GI distress

Metabolic alkalosis

- Disturbed thought processes related to acid-base imbalance
- Ineffective breathing pattern related to hypoventilation
- Risk for injury related to muscle weakness

Multiple myeloma

- Acute pain related to neoplasm that infiltrates the bone
- Fatigue related to illness
- Risk for infection related to immunosuppression

Multiple sclerosis

- Compromised family coping related to effects of progressive, debilitating disease on family members and resultant alteration in role-related behavior patterns
- Constipation related to decreased peristalsis
- Dressing/grooming self-care deficit related to neuromuscular impairment
- Fatigue related to weakness and spasticity
- Impaired physical mobility related to demyelinization
- Impaired verbal communication related to dysarthria
- Interrupted family processes related to role disturbance and uncertain future
- Powerlessness related to remissions and exacerbations of illness
- Readiness for enhanced comfort related to acceptance of care and support of significant others
- Risk for injury related to:
  – gait impairment
  – vertigo
  – vision disturbances
- Sexual dysfunction related to fatigue, decreased sensation, muscle spasm, or urinary incontinence
- Situational low self-esteem related to progressive, debilitating effects of disease
- Urinary retention related to sensorimotor deficits

Myasthenia gravis

- Activity intolerance related to muscle fatigue and weakness
- Dressing/grooming self care deficit related to neuromuscular involvement
- Fatigue related to muscle weakness
- Impaired swallowing related to cerebellar dysfunction
- Ineffective airway clearance related to impaired ability to cough
- Ineffective therapeutic regimen management related to insufficient knowledge of disease
- Risk for injury related to vision disturbance and weakness
- Risk for spiritual distress related to chronic illness
- Risk for urge urinary incontinence related to neuromuscular involvement

Myocardial infarction

- Activity intolerance related to weakness and fatigue
- Acute pain (chest) related to decreased myocardial oxygenation
- Death anxiety related to diagnosis
- Decreased cardiac output related to altered heart rate, rhythm

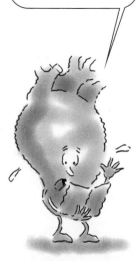

Says here that patients can experience death anxiety related to a diagnosis of myocardial infarction. Yikes!

- Deficient knowledge (diagnostic procedures, therapeutic interventions, and long-range implications for lifestyle changes) related to complex diagnosis and therapeutic regimen
- Impaired gas exchange related to ventilation-perfusion imbalance
- Ineffective coping related to fear of death, anxiety, denial, or depression
- Risk for constipation related to diet, bed rest, or medications
- Risk for injury related to myocardial ischemia, injury, necrosis, inflammation, or arrhythmias

Myocarditis

- Activity intolerance related to weakness and fatigue
- Decreased cardiac output related to arrhythmias
- Fatigue related to infection

Nephrectomy

- Acute pain related to surgical procedure
- Ineffective airway clearance related to:
  – anesthesia
  – immobility
  – location of incision
  – pain
  – presence of chest tube
- Risk for imbalanced fluid volume related to decreased renal reserve and third-space fluid shifting immediately after surgery
- Risk for perioperative positioning related to flank positioning and outermost arm positioning

Nephrotic syndrome

- Imbalanced nutrition: Less than body requirements related to high-protein, low-sodium diet
- Risk for imbalanced fluid volume related to disease process
- Risk for infection related to immunosuppression

Neuritis, peripheral

- Disturbed sensory perception (tactile) related to degeneration of peripheral nerves
- Impaired physical mobility related to muscle weakness
- Risk for injury related to disturbed sensory perception

Neurogenic bladder

- Reflex urinary incontinence related to neuromuscular dysfunction of the lower urinary tract
- Risk for compromised human dignity related to incontinence
- Risk for infection related to incomplete emptying of bladder

Obesity

- Activity intolerance related to deconditioned status and excessive energy demands secondary to obesity
- Disturbed body image related to social stigma of obesity
- Imbalanced nutrition: More than body requirements related to:
  - dysfunctional eating patterns
  - energy expenditure imbalance
  - excess food intake
  - inherited disposition
  - sedentary activity level
- Impaired gas exchange related to ventilation-perfusion imbalance
- Impaired physical mobility related to fatigue with minimal exertion, joint or back discomfort, limitation of motion from extra skin folds
- Risk for impaired skin integrity related to:
  - altered circulation (edema)
  - multiple moist skin folds
  - nutritional deficit
- Social isolation related to size too large for standard seating and body image disturbance

Osteoarthritis

- Activity intolerance related to pain
- Chronic pain related to deterioration of joint cartilage
- Impaired home maintenance related to inadequate support systems, decreased range of motion with increased joint pain

Osteomyelitis

- Acute pain related to inflammation
- Deficient knowledge (prolonged treatment regimen for infection and measures to prevent recurrence) related to new diagnosis
- Impaired physical mobility related to pain
- Risk for disuse syndrome related to prolonged infection, pain, and immobilization
- Risk for injury related to use of antibiotics with high potential for toxic effects

Osteoporosis

- Anxiety related to change in health status
- Disturbed body image related to joint deformity
- Ineffective sexuality patterns related to pain
- Risk for trauma related to bone loss

Otosclerosis

- Deficient knowledge (disease) related to lack of exposure to information
- Disturbed sensory perception (auditory) related to decreased motion of bones of the middle ear
- Risk for infection related to surgery

Ovarian cancer

- Constipation related to GI obstruction
- Deficient knowledge (disease and treatment options) related to lack of exposure to information
- Grieving related to potential loss
- Urinary retention related to obstruction

Ovarian cyst

- Acute pain related to complications of ovarian cysts that cause acute abdominal symptoms
- Anxiety related to laparoscopic surgery
- Ineffective sexuality patterns related to irregular or prolonged bleeding

Paget's disease

- Acute pain related to impingement of abnormal bone on spinal cord
- Bathing/hygiene, dressing/grooming, toileting self-care deficit related to musculoskeletal impairment
- Disturbed body image related to musculoskeletal impairment
- Impaired physical mobility related to asymmetrical bowing of tibia and femur

Pancreatic cancer

- Acute pain related to tumor pressure
- Anxiety related to threat of death and disease status
- Caregiver role strain related to illness severity
- Imbalanced nutrition: Less than body requirements related to:
  - impaired digestion
  - loss of appetite
  - pain
  - vomiting

Pancreatitis

- Acute pain related to:
  - abscess formation or hemorrhaging
  - autodigestive processes and necrosis
  - edema of the pancreas and surrounding tissues
  - peritonitis
- Imbalanced nutrition: Less than body requirements related to:
  - gastric suction
  - impaired digestion
  - nothing-by-mouth status
  - vomiting
- Nausea related to gastric distention
- Risk for deficient fluid volume related to:
  - fluid shifts
  - hemorrhage
  - hyperglycemia
  - vomiting
- Risk for infection related to trauma and chronic disease
- Risk for injury related to:
  - alcoholism
  - hypovolemia
  - pulmonary insults

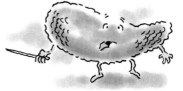

Watch patients
with pancreatitis for
signs of imbalanced
nutrition. I'm feeling
queasy just looking
at this list.

Parkinson's disease

- Activity intolerance related to neuromuscular impairment
- Bathing/hygiene, dressing/grooming self-care deficit related to neuromuscular impairment
- Impaired home maintenance related to disease effects
- Risk for aspiration related to impaired muscles of swallowing
- Risk for falls related to impaired gait and balance

Pelvic inflammatory disease

- Acute pain related to inflammation
- Risk for infection related to inadequate primary defenses
- Sexual dysfunction related to malaise and profuse, purulent vaginal discharge

Peptic ulcers

- Acute pain related to ulcers
- Deficient knowledge (ulcer prevention and care) related to lack of exposure to information
- Nausea related to GI distress

Percutaneous transluminal coronary angioplasty

- Acute pain related to restrictions on mobility and percutaneous puncture at groin site

- Anxiety related to known risks associated with the procedure
- Deficient knowledge (postdischarge care) related to lack of exposure to information
- Risk for injury related to break in skin and presence of foreign body intravascularly

Pericarditis

- Acute pain related to inflammation of pericardium
- Decreased cardiac output related to pericarditis
- Ineffective tissue perfusion (cardiopulmonary) related to decreased cellular exchange

Peripheral vascular disease

- Activity intolerance related to pain
- Impaired physical mobility related to pain and activity intolerance
- Impaired tissue integrity (peripheral) related to decreased oxygenation
- Risk for peripheral neurovascular dysfunction related to vascular obstruction

Perirectal abscess and fistula

- Acute pain related to abscess and fistula
- Delayed surgical recovery related to inflammation
- Situational low self-esteem related to difficult healing process

Peritonitis

- Acute pain related to inflammation
- Nausea related to increased GI pressure
- Risk for infection related to inadequate primary defenses

Permanent pacemaker insertion

- Bathing/hygiene self-care deficit related to bed rest and activity limitations
- Deficient knowledge (self-care after discharge) related to unfamiliar therapeutic intervention
- Disturbed body image related to dependence on pacemaker
- Risk for infection related to surgical disruption of skin barrier

Pituitary tumor

- Acute pain related to tumor pressure
- Deficient knowledge (surgical options) related to lack of exposure to information
- Disturbed sensory perception (visual) related to unilateral blindness
- Risk for injury related to dementia

Pleural effusion and empyema

- Fatigue related to weakness
- Hyperthermia related to infection
- Ineffective breathing pattern related to pain and increased work of breathing

Pleurisy

- Acute pain related to inflammation of visceral and parietal pleurae
- Impaired gas exchange related to altered oxygen supply
- Ineffective breathing pattern related limited movement on affected side

Pneumocystis carinii pneumonia

- Fatigue related to infection
- Grieving related to poor prognosis
- Ineffective breathing pattern related to fatigue
- Risk for imbalanced body temperature related to infection

Pneumonia

- Acute pain related to fever and pleuritic irritation
- Bathing/hygiene self-care deficit related to weakness and tiredness
- Deficient fluid volume related to active fluid volume loss
- Deficient knowledge (treatment regimen) related to lack of exposure to information
- Impaired gas exchange related to ventilation-perfusion imbalance
- Ineffective airway clearance related to retained secretions
- Risk for infection related to stress and other risk factors

Pneumothorax

- Acute pain related to air trapped in the intrapleural space
- Fear related to sudden onset of illness
- Impaired gas exchange related to ventilation-perfusion imbalance
- Ineffective tissue perfusion (cardiopulmonary) related to collapsed lung

Polycystic kidney disease

- Acute pain related to kidney mass
- Deficient knowledge (illness) related to lack of exposure to information
- Ineffective tissue perfusion (renal) related to kidney mass

Polycythemia vera

- Acute pain related to headache
- Deficient knowledge (disease and treatment) related to lack of exposure to information
- Disturbed sensory perception (visual) related to hypervolemia
- Impaired gas exchange related to dyspnea

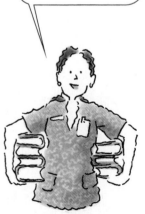

Lack of exposure to information can lead to deficient knowledge about an illness. I thought I might do a little reading about polycystic kidney disease.

Potassium imbalance

- Decreased cardiac output related to arrhythmias
- Diarrhea related to hypercalcemia and hypocalcemia
- Nausea related to GI distress

Pressure ulcers

- Imbalanced nutrition: Less than body requirements related to inability to digest and absorb nutrients
- Impaired physical mobility related to musculoskeletal and neuromuscular impairment
- Impaired skin integrity related to:
  – altered circulation
  – altered sensation
  – impaired physical mobility
  – mechanical factors
- Risk for infection related to impaired skin integrity

Prostatectomy

- Acute pain related to:
  – bladder spasms
  – catheter obstruction
  – surgical intervention
  – urethral stricture
- Risk for deficient fluid volume related to prostatic or incisional bleeding after surgery
- Risk for infection (postoperative) related to:
  – abdominal drain placement
  – preoperative status
  – urinary catheter
- Risk for situational low self-esteem related to:
  – incontinence
  – potential impotence
  – sexual alterations
- Sexual dysfunction (decreased libido) related to:
  – decreased self-esteem
  – fear of incontinence
  – impotence related to parasympathetic nerve damage (from radical prostatectomy)
  – infertility related to retrograde ejaculation (from transurethral resection of the prostate and suprapubic prostatectomy)
- Urge urinary incontinence related to:
  – decrease in detrusor muscle
  – sphincter tone
  – trauma to the bladder neck
  – urinary catheter removal
- Urinary retention related to urinary catheter obstruction

Prostatic cancer

- Acute pain related to physical, biological, or chemical agents
- Anxiety related to change in health status
- Sexual dysfunction related to impotence
- Urinary retention related to obstruction

Prostatitis

- Acute pain related to infection and destruction of tissue
- Hyperthermia related to infection
- Impaired urinary elimination related to infection

Pseudomembranous enterocolitis

- Deficient fluid volume related to active loss
- Diarrhea related to inflammation
- Impaired skin integrity related to severe diarrhea

Psoriasis

- Disturbed body image related to itchy, dry, cracked, and encrusted lesions on body parts
- Impaired skin integrity related to itchy, dry, cracked, and encrusted lesions
- Social isolation related to disturbed body image

Pulmonary edema

- Decreased cardiac output related to tachycardia
- Dysfunctional ventilatory weaning response related to anxiety
- Excess fluid volume related to fluid accumulation in extravascular spaces of the lungs
- Ineffective breathing pattern related to diminished lung compliance

Pulmonary embolism and infarction

- Activity intolerance related to imbalance between oxygen supply and demand
- Acute pain related to biological injury
- Compromised family coping related to potentially life-threatening situation
- Decreased cardiac output related to altered heart rate and rhythm
- Deficient fluid volume related to active fluid volume loss
- Deficient knowledge (treatment regimen) related to complex disorder and therapy
- Impaired gas exchange related to ventilation-perfusion mismatch

Pulmonary hypertension

- Bathing/hygiene, dressing/grooming self-care deficit related to fatigue
- Decreased cardiac output related to altered heart rate and rhythm
- Ineffective breathing pattern related to hypertrophy of small pulmonary arteries
- Ineffective tissue perfusion (cardiopulmonary) related to impaired transport of oxygen across alveolar and capillary membranes

Pyelonephritis

- Excess fluid volume related to compromised regulatory mechanisms
- Hyperthermia related to infection
- Impaired urinary elimination related to urgency, burning, or nocturia
- Risk for infection related to inadequate primary and secondary defenses

Radioactive implant for cervical cancer

- Ineffective sexuality patterns related to vaginal tissue changes or fear of radioactivity
- Risk for disuse syndrome related to imposed bed rest
- Risk for injury related to dislodgment of the implant

Rape-trauma syndrome

- Rape-trauma syndrome related to rape or attempted rape
- Rape-trauma syndrome: Compound reaction related to rape
- Rape-trauma syndrome: Silent reaction related to rape
- Situational low self-esteem related to rape

Raynaud's disease

- Disturbed sensory perception (tactile) related to decreased oxygenation
- Ineffective tissue perfusion (peripheral) related to decreased arterial blood flow
- Risk for impaired skin integrity related to decreased sensation and ischemia

Patients with Raynaud's disease are at risk for impaired skin integrity related to decreased sensation. Is it cold in here, or is it just me?

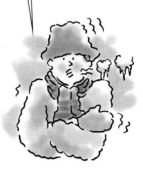

Renal calculi

- Acute pain related to obstruction of ureter or kidney by renal calculi
- Deficient knowledge (disease) related to lack of exposure to information
- Risk for infection related to trauma
- Urinary retention related to ureter obstruction by renal calculi

Renal dialysis

- Acute pain related to hemodialysis treatment
- Imbalanced nutrition: Less than body requirements related to:
  - abdominal distention
  - anorexia
  - nausea
  - stomatitis
- Impaired physical mobility related to lengthy treatment regimen
- Ineffective breathing pattern related to elevation of diaphragm during peritoneal dialysis exchanges and reduced mobility
- Risk for acute confusion related to consequences of long-term dialysis treatment
- Risk for fluid imbalance related to dialysis
- Risk for infection related to invasive procedure
- Risk for injury related to:
  - bleeding from the area around the vascular access device
  - potential for thrombosis, stenosis, or hematoma of vascular access
- Risk for injury (perforation or ileus) related to catheter insertion or irritation from dialysate

Renal failure, acute

- Deficient knowledge (acute renal failure and dialysis) related to lack of exposure to information on complex disease and its management
- Excess fluid volume related to sodium and water retention
- Imbalanced nutrition: Less than body requirements related to anorexia, nausea and vomiting, and restricted dietary intake
- Impaired urinary elimination related to disease process
- Risk for infection related to decreased immune response and skin changes secondary to uremia
- Risk for injury related to uremic syndrome

Renal failure, chronic

- Caregiver role strain related to illness chronicity
- Chronic low self-esteem related to chronic disease
- Disturbed thought processes related to:
  - acidosis
  - fluid and electrolyte imbalances
  - uremic toxins
- Excess fluid volume related to fluid retention
- Imbalanced nutrition: Less than body requirements related to:
  - altered metabolism of proteins, lipids, and carbohydrates
  - anorexia
  - diarrhea
  - GI inflammation with poor absorption
  - nausea and vomiting
  - restricted dietary intake

- Impaired oral mucous membrane related to accumulation of urea and ammonia
- Noncompliance (treatment regimen) related to:
  - deficient knowledge
  - denial
  - lack of resources
  - lack of social support systems
- Risk for impaired skin integrity related to:
  - abnormal blood clotting
  - anemia
  - calcium phosphate deposits on the skin
  - capillary fragility
  - decreased activity of oil and sweat glands
  - retention of pigments
  - scratching
- Sexual dysfunction related to the effects of uremia on the endocrine system and central nervous system and to the psychosocial impact of chronic renal failure and its treatment

Respiratory acidosis

- Decreased cardiac output related to altered heart rate and rhythm
- Impaired gas exchange related to ventilatory-perfusion imbalance
- Ineffective breathing pattern related to hypoventilation

Respiratory alkalosis

- Anxiety related to hyperventilation
- Impaired gas exchange related to ventilatory-perfusion imbalance
- Ineffective breathing pattern related to hyperventilation

Retinal detachment

- Disturbed sensory perception (visual) related to loosening of retina
- Impaired physical mobility related to vision disturbance
- Ineffective coping related to decreased vision and impending surgery

Rheumatoid arthritis

- Activity intolerance related to pain and swelling of joints
- Chronic pain related to inflammation of joints
- Disturbed body image related to arthritic joints
- Ineffective health maintenance related to lack of mobility

Salmonellosis

- Diarrhea related to GI distress
- Hyperthermia related to infection
- Risk for deficient fluid volume related to diarrhea

Sarcoidosis

- Activity intolerance related to pain
- Decreased cardiac output related to arrhythmias
- Deficient knowledge (disease and treatment) related to lack of exposure to information
- Ineffective breathing pattern related to pain

Scabies

- Impaired skin integrity related to skin infection
- Ineffective sexual patterns related to fear of spreading infection
- Social isolation related to fear of spreading infection

Seizure disorder

- Acute confusion related to postictal state
- Deficient knowledge (seizure management) related to lack of exposure to information
- Impaired memory related to neurologic disturbance
- Ineffective airway clearance related to:
  - airway occlusion by tongue or foreign body
  - apnea
  - excessive secretions
  - jaw clenching
  - loss of consciousness
- Ineffective therapeutic regimen management related to deficient knowledge of disease, seizure care, and community resources
- Risk for injury related to excessive uncontrolled muscle activity
- Risk for trauma related to internal factors

Septic arthritis

- Acute pain related to inflammation of joints
- Anxiety related to threat to health and roles
- Risk for infection related to inadequate primary and secondary defenses

Septic shock

- Acute confusion related to decreased cerebral tissue perfusion
- Diarrhea related to GI irritation
- Hyperthermia related to infection
- Imbalanced nutrition: Less than body requirements related to inadequate intake and active fluid and nutrient loss
- Impaired gas exchange related to ventilation-perfusion imbalance and diffusion defects
- Ineffective coping related to threat to life
- Risk for injury due to complications related to ischemia or bleeding

Sinusitis

- Acute pain related to inflammation and pressure
- Fatigue related to infection
- Risk for infection related to inadequate primary defenses

Sjögren's syndrome

- Disturbed sensory perception (visual) related to ocular dryness
- Fatigue related to disease process
- Impaired oral mucous membrane related to oral dryness

Skin grafts

- Deficient knowledge (home care of donor and graft sites) related to lack of exposure to information
- Disturbed body image related to wound and potential scarring
- Imbalanced nutrition: Less than body requirements related to increased metabolic needs secondary to tissue healing
- Impaired physical mobility related to position and movement limitations
- Risk for infection of donor site related to surgical excision

Spinal cord injury

- Bathing/hygiene, dressing/grooming, feeding, toileting self-care deficit related to spinal cord injury
- Constipation related to loss of voluntary bowel control
- Decreased cardiac output related to autonomic dysfunction and immobility
- Deficient diversional activity related to loss of mobility or function
- Disturbed body image related to physical disability
- Imbalanced nutrition: Less than body requirements related to acute injury
- Impaired gas exchange related to loss of use of phrenic nerve, intercostal muscles, or abdominal muscles secondary to the spinal injury
- Impaired home maintenance related to inadequate support systems
- Impaired physical mobility related to muscular paralysis
- Impaired urinary elimination related to interruption of neural innervation
- Incontinence, bowel and total urinary related to neuromuscular enervation
- Ineffective airway clearance related to loss of use of intercostal muscles
- Risk for autonomic dysreflexia related to damage to spinal cord with another associated stressor
- Risk for infection related to catheterization

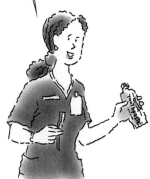

Spinal cord injuries can cause many deficits related to self-care. Brush up on the ones listed here.

Spinal neoplasm

- Impaired physical mobility related to neuromuscular impairment
- Incontinence, bowel and total urinary related to neurologic dysfunction
- Risk for autonomic dysreflexia related to spinal cord injury or lesion
- Risk for impaired skin integrity related to:
  - altered nutritional status
  - altered sensation
  - mechanical factors
  - moisture from incontinence
  - physical immobilization

Squamous cell carcinoma

- Anxiety related to threat to health status
- Impaired skin integrity related to invasive tumor of skin
- Ineffective therapeutic regimen management related to deficient knowledge

Stomatitis

- Acute pain related to swollen and easily bruised gums and mucous membranes
- Impaired oral mucous membrane related to:
  - chemical irritants
  - infection
  - malnutrition or vitamin deficiency
  - mechanical irritants (ill-fitting dentures, braces)
- Risk for infection related to immunosuppression

Stroke

- Bathing/hygiene, dressing/grooming, feeding, toileting self-care deficit related to:
  - neuromuscular impairment
  - perceptual cognitive impairment
  - weakness or lack of motivation
- Caregiver role strain related to increased care needs
- Chronic confusion related to cerebral injury
- Deficient knowledge (stroke management) related to lack of exposure to information on self-care
- Impaired physical mobility related to damage to motor cortex or motor pathways
- Impaired verbal communication related to cerebral injury
- Ineffective airway clearance related to hemiplegic effects of a stroke
- Ineffective tissue perfusion (cerebral) related to clot or hemorrhage

- Risk for disuse syndrome related to neuromuscular impairment
- Unilateral neglect related to cerebral injury

Syphilis

- Ineffective coping related to situational crisis
- Ineffective sexuality patterns related to fear of spreading illness
- Risk for infection related to external factors

Tendinitis and bursitis

- Activity intolerance related to pain and stiffness
- Acute pain related to inflammation
- Ineffective role performance related to restricted movement of joint due to pain

Thoracotomy

- Acute pain related to surgical incision
- Deficient knowledge (treatment regimen) related to unfamiliarity with thoracotomy
- Impaired gas exchange related to:
  – analgesic medications
  – atelectasis
  – hypoventilation from anesthesia
  – pain
  – thickened secretions
- Risk for infection related to surgical incision and endotracheal intubation

Thrombocytopenia

- Decreased cardiac output related to tachycardia
- Deficient knowledge (disease and treatment) related to lack of exposure to information
- Fatigue related to disease process
- Risk for injury related to possible bleeding from lack of platelets

Thrombophlebitis

- Acute pain related to vessel obstruction and edema
- Deficient knowledge (treatment regimen) related to lack of exposure to information
- Ineffective tissue perfusion (peripheral) related to interruption of venous flow

Thyroid cancer

- Deficient knowledge (treatment regimen) related to lack of exposure to information
- Impaired swallowing related to pressure of thyroid nodule
- Ineffective breathing pattern related to enlarged thyroid nodule

Toxic shock syndrome

- Diarrhea related to infection
- Fear related to sudden onset of illness
- Hyperthermia related to infection

Tracheostomy

- Impaired skin integrity related to humidity, moisture, or mucus accumulation
- Ineffective breathing pattern related to tracheal tube dislodgment or plugging
- Risk for aspiration related to impaired swallowing and vomiting
- Risk for injury (poor oxygenation) related to suctioning procedure

Trauma

- Impaired gas exchange related to:
  - head injury
  - pulmonary injury
  - shock
- Impaired physical mobility related to orthopedic injury
- Risk for imbalanced fluid volume related to hypovolemia or cardiac injury
- Risk for injury (complications) related to:
  - hypermetabolic state
  - impaired immunologic defenses
  - stress
- Risk for posttrauma syndrome related to perception of event and sudden, unexpected injury

Trigeminal neuralgia

- Acute pain related to disorder of the fifth cranial nerve
- Anxiety related to threat to health
- Ineffective coping related to inadequate level of perception of control

Tuberculosis

- Deficient knowledge (disease process) related to lack of exposure to information
- Ineffective airway clearance related to tracheobronchial obstruction or secretions
- Ineffective breathing pattern related to decreased energy or fatigue
- Risk for infection related to altered primary defenses
- Social isolation related to fear of spreading disease

Trigeminal neuralgia can cause acute pain. What nerve!

Ulcerative colitis

- Anxiety related to change in health status
- Diarrhea related to inflammation of colon
- Fatigue related to loss of fluids and diarrhea
- Imbalanced nutrition: Less than body requirements related to inability to absorb nutrients
- Ineffective role performance related to frequent diarrhea

Urinary tract infection

- Acute pain related to inflammation and muscle spasms
- Deficient knowledge (disease process) related to lack of exposure to information
- Impaired urinary elimination related to obstruction

Urolithiasis

- Acute pain related to:
  - incision
  - passage of calculus fragments
  - procedural manipulation
- Deficient knowledge (potential causes of calculus formation) related to lack of exposure to information
- Impaired urinary elimination: Dysuria, oliguria, pyuria, or frequency related to:
  - calculus fragment passage
  - hematuria
  - infection
  - obstruction

Uterine cancer

- Acute pain related to cancer
- Imbalanced nutrition: Less than body requirements related to cancer
- Spiritual distress related to chronic illness

Uterine prolapse

- Anxiety related to change in health status
- Disturbed body image related to biophysical factors
- Stress urinary incontinence related to weak pelvic musculature

Valvular heart disease

- Activity intolerance related to fatigue and dyspnea on exertion
- Anxiety related to change in health status
- Decreased cardiac output related to mechanical disruption
- Ineffective breathing pattern related to decreased energy and fatigue

Vascular retinopathy

- Disturbed sensory perception (visual) related to disturbed blood supply to the eye
- Ineffective coping related to chronic illness
- Risk for injury related to loss of vision

Vasculitis

- Disturbed body image related to illness
- Imbalanced nutrition: Less than body requirements related to anorexia of disease process
- Ineffective tissue perfusion (cerebral, cardiopulmonary, gastrointestinal, renal, peripheral) related to inflamed vessels causing impaired blood flow to nearby organs
- Risk for infection related to impaired defenses

Vulvovaginitis

- Acute pain related to inflammation
- Ineffective sexuality patterns related to vaginal inflammation, itching, and irritation
- Risk for infection related to inadequate primary defenses

Wounds

- Acute pain related to trauma to nerve endings
- Impaired skin integrity related to penetration of skin
- Risk for contamination related to detrimental home environmental factors
- Risk for deficient fluid volume related to active loss from trauma
- Risk for infection related to inadequate primary defenses

Maternal-neonatal diagnoses

Just the facts

In this chapter, you'll learn:

♦ nursing diagnoses that correlate with common maternal-neonatal medical diagnoses.

A look at maternal-neonatal diagnoses

This chapter covers medical diagnoses that are applicable to pregnant patients and their neonates. Maternal-neonatal care can be complex because both the mother and neonate have many needs. The diagnoses listed here are just a sampling of the diagnoses that you might encounter on a maternity unit. Each entry provides a list of a few of the major nursing diagnoses and related factors to be considered after your assessment. Remember that the nursing diagnoses listed here represent the needs most commonly associated with the medical condition; your patient may have different needs.

> Maternal-neonatal care must address the needs of both the mother and the neonate.

Abortion

- Anxiety related to situational crisis or unmet needs
- Complicated grieving related to loss of fetus
- Risk for deficient fluid volume related to bleeding

Abruptio placentae

- Acute pain related to separation of placenta
- Deficient fluid volume related to bleeding
- Grieving related to potential loss of fetus
- Ineffective tissue perfusion (cardiopulmonary of neonate) related to decreased cellular exchange

Acquired immunodeficiency syndrome—Infant

- Fear (parent) related to infant's future death as a result of human immunodeficiency virus (HIV) infection
- Risk for infection related to perinatal transmission of HIV and immunosuppression
- Risk for injury related to transmission of HIV to personnel and other infants in the nursery

Cardiovascular disease in pregnancy

- Activity intolerance related to heart failure
- Decreased cardiac output related to heart decompensation and arrhythmias
- Risk for imbalanced fluid volume related to compromised regulatory mechanism

Cesarean birth

- Activity intolerance related to:
  - anesthetic administration
  - delivery
  - pain
  - surgical incision
- Acute pain related to surgical incision
- Ineffective coping related to surgical intervention, perceived loss of the birthing experience, and fatigue
- Risk for deficient fluid volume related to bleeding associated with surgery
- Risk for infection (maternal) related surgical incision, repeated vaginal examination, sequelae of anesthetic administration, bladder intubation, or I.V. lines

Choanal atresia

- Disabled family coping related to:
  - anxiety
  - emotional conflict as a result of infant's defect
  - guilt
- Ineffective breathing pattern related to obstruction from congenital defect

Diabetes-related complications during pregnancy

- Imbalanced nutrition: More than body requirements related to altered carbohydrate metabolism

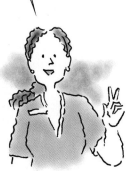

Two diabetes-related complications associated with ineffective breathing patterns are uterine enlargement and excessive amniotic fluid.

- Ineffective breathing pattern related to uterine enlargement and excessive amniotic fluid
- Risk for infection related to disease process
- Risk for injury (fetal) related to dependence on maternal glycemic states

Drug addiction and withdrawal

- Deficient knowledge (safe, healthy neonatal care and development) related to emotional inadequacy and lack of exposure to information about infant care
- Imbalanced nutrition: Less than body requirements related to:
  – poor or low intake because of lack of coordination in sucking or swallowing
  – vomiting
- Ineffective coping (maternal) related to drug abuse or inability to care for the infant
- Ineffective infant feeding pattern related to delayed neurologic development
- Risk for deficient fluid volume related to diarrhea or vomiting
- Risk for impaired skin integrity related to perianal irritation from diarrhea and rubbing against sheets because of hyperactivity
- Risk for injury (respiratory and neurologic) related to withdrawal from drug exposure

Ectopic pregnancy

- Acute pain related to disruption of pelvic tissue
- Deficient fluid volume related to bleeding
- Fear related to loss of pregnancy and threat to fertility
- Risk for infection related to the trauma of tubal rupture and peritoneal inflammation

Fetal alcohol syndrome

- Deficient knowledge (parental) related to lack of information about infant care
- Delayed growth and development related to neurologic and mental deficiency
- Dysfunctional family processes: Alcoholism related to abuse of alcohol
- Imbalanced nutrition: Less than body requirements related to lack of nutritional reserves and to poor intake
- Risk for impaired parenting related to previous lifestyle associated with alcohol abuse or to unrealistic expectations of self and infant

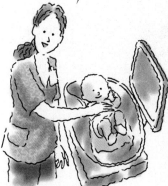

Fetal alcohol syndrome can cause delays in growth and development.

Hydrocephalus

- Anxiety (parent and child) related to lack of understanding about the child's condition and treatment
- Compromised family coping related to illness of baby
- Delayed growth and development related to disease
- Excess fluid volume related to placement of ventriculoatrial shunt
- Imbalanced nutrition: Less than body requirements related to feeding difficulties
- Ineffective tissue perfusion (cerebral) related to increased intracranial pressure
- Risk for deficient fluid volume related to altered nutritional status in the preoperative and postoperative phases
- Risk for infection related to surgical placement of shunt
- Risk for injury related to onset of seizures

Hyperemesis gravidarum

- Acute pain related to repeated episodes of vomiting
- Deficient fluid volume related to protracted emesis
- Fear related to hospitalization and pregnancy outcome
- Imbalanced nutrition: Less than body requirements related to nausea and vomiting and subsequent inconsistent or insufficient food intake

Hypertension, pregnancy induced

- Deficient knowledge (signs and symptoms of increased blood pressure) related to lack of exposure
- Excess fluid volume related to compromised regulatory mechanism
- Risk for injury (fetal) related to impaired maternal-placental perfusion
- Risk for injury (maternal) related to organ or system dysfunction as a sequela of vasospasm and increased blood pressure

Hysterectomy

- Acute pain related to abdominal incision and distention
- Disturbed body image related to changes in body appearance and function as a result of surgery
- Sexual dysfunction (decreased libido or dyspareunia) related to:
  - altered body image
  - concerns about acceptance by spouse or partner
  - decreased estrogen levels
  - fatigue
  - grieving
  - loss of vaginal sensations
  - pain
  - sexual activity restrictions

- Urinary retention related to decreased bladder and urethral muscle tone from anesthesia and mechanical trauma

Mastitis and breast engorgement

- Acute pain related to inflammation and milk engorgement
- Risk for imbalanced body temperature related to infection
- Risk for infection related to inadequate primary defenses

Meconium aspiration syndrome

- Disabled family coping related to anxiety and guilt
- Ineffective breathing pattern related to meconium aspiration

Multiple gestation

- Ineffective coping related to dramatic increase in family size
- Risk for injury (maternal and fetal) related to physiologic demands of a multifetal pregnancy
- Risk for injury related to preterm labor and delivery

Myelomeningocele

- Constipation related to level of spinal cord injury
- Delayed growth and development related to the hospital stay
- Hypothermia related to heat loss through the sac
- Imbalanced nutrition: Less than body requirements related to surgery
- Impaired skin integrity related to presence of sac and surgical procedure
- Impaired urinary elimination related to injury of spinal cord nerves
- Ineffective tissue perfusion (cerebral) related to hydrocephalus and increased intracranial pressure
- Risk for impaired parenting related to separation from the infant at birth
- Risk for impaired skin integrity related to contact with urine or feces and altered mobility

Necrotizing enterocolitis

- Diarrhea related to inflammation
- Ineffective infant feeding pattern related to nothing-by-mouth status
- Interrupted family processes related to shift in health status of family member

Neural tube defects

- Decisional conflict (possible abortion) related to genetic defect
- Interrupted family processes related to change in health status of family member
- Spiritual distress related to chronic illness

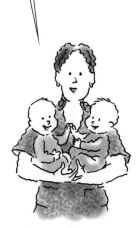

A dramatic increase in family size can lead to ineffective coping. Sure, these two can be a handful, but imagine trying to juggle quadruplets.

Placenta previa

- Anxiety related to unknown hospital procedures
- Deficient fluid volume related to active loss, bleeding
- Fear related to unknown fetal outcome
- Risk for injury (fetal) related to uteroplacental insufficiency

Premature rupture of membranes

- Anxiety related to situational crisis
- Risk for infection related to lack of primary defenses

Puerperal infection

- Acute pain related to inflammatory processes and exudate entrapment
- Anxiety related to threat to health status
- Risk for infection related to the trauma of labor, delivery, and the iatrogenic introduction of pathogens

Respiratory distress syndrome

- Decreased cardiac output related to disease
- Disabled family coping related to anxiety, guilt, and separation from the infant as a result of situational crisis
- Imbalanced nutrition: Less than body requirements related to:
  - decreased gastric motility
  - inability to ingest feedings
  - withholding of food and water
- Impaired gas exchange related to:
  - alveolar ventilation
  - lung perfusion
  - reduced lung volume and compliance
- Risk for deficient fluid volume related to active fluid losses
- Risk for injury related to medical therapy and treatments

Toxoplasmosis

- Deficient knowledge (treatment regimen) related to lack of exposure to information
- Fatigue related to localized infection
- Hyperthermia related to infection

Pediatric diagnoses

Just the facts

In this chapter, you'll learn:

♦ nursing diagnoses that correlate with common pediatric medical diagnoses.

A look at pediatric diagnoses

This chapter covers medical diagnoses that are common in pediatric patients. Remember that pediatric patients can have the same medical and nursing diagnoses as an adult; however, the care provided for these patients may be different. Each entry provides a list of a few of the major nursing diagnoses and related factors to be considered after your assessment. Remember that the nursing diagnoses listed here represent the needs most commonly associated with the medical condition in pediatric patients; your pediatric patient may have different needs.

> Although pediatric patients can have the same diagnoses as adults, the care provided may be different.

Acne vulgaris

- Deficient knowledge (care of skin) related to lack of exposure to information
- Situational low self-esteem related to face lesions
- Social isolation related to alteration in physical appearance

Anorexia nervosa

- Deficient fluid volume related to active loss
- Disturbed body image related to psychological effects of the disorder
- Imbalanced nutrition: Less than body requirements related to fear of obesity
- Impaired social interaction related to low self-esteem
- Interrupted family processes related to illness of family member
- Social isolation related to eating habits

Aplastic and hypoplastic anemias

- Fatigue related to disease process
- Ineffective breathing pattern related to weakness and fatigue
- Ineffective family coping related to altered health status of family member
- Risk for infection related to destruction of stem cells in bone marrow

Arm and leg fractures

- Bathing/hygiene, dressing/grooming, feeding self-care deficit related to immobility of affected limb
- Impaired walking related to cast or splints
- Risk for injury related to inability to use body part

Asthma

- Activity intolerance related to imbalance between oxygen supply and demand
- Anxiety related to threat to health status
- Deficient knowledge (home care procedures) related to new diagnosis
- Deficient knowledge (treatment regimen) related to complexity of therapeutic regimen
- Fatigue related to hypoxia
- Impaired gas exchange related to bronchial constriction
- Ineffective airway clearance related to constriction
- Readiness for enhanced management of therapeutic regimen related to perceived benefits
- Risk for deficient fluid volume related to loss of fluid from the respiratory tract

Attention deficit hyperactivity disorder

- Impaired social interaction related to hyperactivity
- Interrupted family processes related to shift in health status of family member
- Risk for delayed development related to brain disorder

Autistic disorder

- Impaired social interaction related to brain disorder
- Impaired verbal communication related to stimulus confusion
- Risk for impaired parenting related to 24-hour demands of child with special needs
- Risk for other-directed or self-directed violence related to impaired capacity to identify and express feelings

Biliary atresia

- Deficient fluid volume related to poor absorption of nutrients
- Deficient knowledge (home care procedures) related to new diagnosis

- Delayed growth and development related to chronic illness

Bronchiolitis

- Anxiety (child and parent) related to lack of knowledge about condition
- Deficient knowledge (home care procedures) related to new diagnosis
- Fatigue related to respiratory distress
- Hyperthermia related to infection
- Imbalanced nutrition: Less than body requirements related to increased metabolic needs
- Impaired gas exchange related to bronchiolar edema and increased mucus production
- Risk for deficient fluid volume related to increased water loss through exhalation and decreased fluid intake
- Social isolation related to isolation precautions

Bronchopulmonary dysplasia

- Anxiety (parent) related to fear and lack of knowledge about the child's illness
- Delayed growth and development related to chronic illness, prematurity, or prolonged hospital stay
- Imbalanced nutrition: Less than body requirements related to increased metabolic rate and high calorie demands
- Impaired gas exchange related to atelectasis
- Risk for impaired parenting related to chronic illness
- Risk for impaired skin integrity related to irritation from nasogastric tube feedings

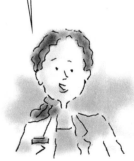

Involuntary movements and impaired muscle function associated with cerebral palsy can lead to deficits in self-care skills.

Bulimia nervosa

- Constipation related to poor eating habits and insufficient fluid intake
- Deficient fluid volume related to active loss
- Disturbed body image related to illness
- Disturbed personal identity related to body weight
- Imbalanced nutrition: Less than body requirements related to binge-purge behavior

Cerebral palsy

- Bathing/hygiene, dressing/grooming, feeding, toileting self-care deficit related to involuntary movements and impaired muscle function
- Caregiver role strain related to complex needs of care receiver
- Delayed growth and development related to neuromuscular impairment
- Impaired physical mobility related to impaired muscle function
- Impaired swallowing related to impaired muscle function

Child abuse

- Delayed growth and development related to inadequate caregiving
- Impaired parenting related to the abusive parent's inability to attach to or bond with the child
- Ineffective family coping related to personal issues that contribute to child abuse
- Risk for other-directed violence (abusive family member) related to maladaptive behavior

Cleft lip and cleft palate

- Disabled family coping related to the stress of hospitalization (preoperative)
- Imbalanced nutrition: Less than body requirements related to impaired feeding (preoperative)
- Impaired skin integrity related to surgical incision
- Ineffective infant feeding pattern related to deformity
- Risk for aspiration related to ineffective feeding

Clubfoot

- Compromised family coping related to situational crisis
- Deficient knowledge (treatment protocols) related to lack of exposure to information
- Impaired physical mobility related to casting or splinting
- Risk for impaired skin integrity related to casting or splinting
- Risk for injury related to failure to provide appropriate care, leading to complications

Complement deficiency

- Deficient knowledge (treatment options) related to lack of exposure to information
- Disabled family coping related to change in health status of family member
- Risk for infection related to increased susceptibility to infection

Congenital heart defect

- Anxiety (child) related to:
  - immobility
  - intensive care unit environment
  - parental anxiety
  - separation from parents
  - surgery
- Anxiety (parent) related to child's congenital heart defect
- Decreased cardiac output related to disease process and surgical procedure
- Deficient knowledge (preoperative and postoperative care) related to impending surgery

- Risk for infection related to immobility and numerous incisions
- Risk for injury related to:
  – blood loss
  – electric current
  – positioning
  – surgical procedure

Congenital hip dysplasia

- Constipation related to immobility
- Deficient diversional activity related to immobility secondary to traction or spica cast
- Risk for impaired skin integrity related to:
  – immobility
  – spica cast
  – traction
- Risk for infection related to break in skin integrity secondary to traction (if pins are used)
- Risk for injury related to possible mechanical malfunctioning of traction or circulatory compromise

Croup

- Anxiety related to hospital stay and respiratory distress
- Ineffective airway clearance related to laryngeal obstruction
- Ineffective breathing pattern related to upper airway edema and thickened secretions
- Risk for deficient fluid volume related to decreased oral intake
- Risk for infection related to break in primary defenses

Cystic fibrosis

- Anxiety (child) related to respiratory distress and hospital stay
- Anxiety (parent) related to lack of knowledge about the child's condition
- Deficient knowledge (home care procedures) related to complex disorder
- Imbalanced nutrition: Less than body requirements related to reduced absorption of nutrients
- Impaired gas exchange related to increased mucus production
- Parental role conflict related to child's hospitalization
- Risk for delayed development related to illness
- Risk for infection related to increased mucus production

Down syndrome

- Bathing/hygiene, dressing/grooming self-care deficit related to mental retardation
- Interrupted family processes related to chronic illness
- Risk for delayed development related to chromosome abnormality

Epiglottiditis

- Anxiety (parent) related to lack of knowledge concerning the child's condition
- Anxiety and fear (child) related to respiratory distress and hospital stay
- Disabled family coping related to anxiety and fear
- Hyperthermia related to infection
- Impaired swallowing related to inflammation and edema
- Ineffective airway clearance related to inflammation and edema
- Ineffective breathing pattern related to upper airway edema
- Risk for deficient fluid volume related to decreased fluid intake

Esophagitis, corrosive

- Impaired parenting related to:
  - deficient knowledge about injury protection
  - poor home environment
  - presence of stress
- Readiness for enhanced parenting related to willingness to enhance parenting
- Risk for poisoning related to presence of poison within reach of child

Fracture

- Acute pain related to muscle spasm, swelling, or bleeding
- Constipation related to immobility
- Impaired gas exchange related to complications secondary to the fracture and immobility
- Ineffective tissue perfusion (peripheral) related to:
  - bleeding
  - swelling
  - the cast
  - traction
- Risk for activity intolerance related to immobility from cast or traction
- Risk for impaired skin integrity related to immobility from cast or traction

Fragile X syndrome

- Delayed growth and development related to X-linked dominant gene inheritance
- Impaired verbal communication related to mental retardation
- Interrupted family processes related to shift in health status of family member
- Risk for caregiver role strain related to complex care needs of care receiver

Glycogen storage disease

- Anxiety (parent) related to lack of knowledge concerning the child's condition
- Delayed growth and development related to chronic illness
- Readiness for enhanced nutrition related to readiness to manage disease through diet

Haemophilus influenzae infection

- Deficient fluid volume related to active loss
- Hyperthermia related to infection
- Impaired gas exchange related to ventilation-perfusion imbalance

Head injury

- Acute pain related to head injury
- Anxiety (child and parent) related to traumatic head injury
- Decreased cardiac output related to hemorrhage
- Deficient knowledge (home care procedures) related to new diagnosis
- Ineffective breathing pattern (with potential for respiratory failure) related to increased intracranial pressure (ICP)
- Ineffective tissue perfusion (peripheral) related to hypotension secondary to hypovolemic shock
- Risk for deficient fluid volume related to nausea and vomiting
- Risk for impaired skin integrity related to physical immobility
- Risk for infection related to injury
- Risk for injury related to altered level of consciousness secondary to head injury or increased ICP (or both)
- Risk for injury secondary to seizures

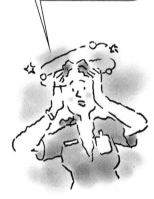

Traumatic head injury can cause anxiety for both the child and the parent. What if my head never stops spinning?

Hemophilia

- Acute pain related to bleeding and swelling
- Chronic low self-esteem related to chronic illness and hospital stay
- Compromized family coping related to repeated hospital stays and the child's chronic illness
- Impaired physical mobility related to decreased range of motion secondary to bleeding and swelling
- Risk for injury (hemorrhage) related to disease

Hirschsprung's disease

- Anxiety (parent) related to lack of knowledge about the disease and prescribed treatment
- Constipation related to aganglionosis
- Disturbed body image related to colostomy or ileostomy
- Impaired skin integrity related to exposure to stools secondary to colostomy or ileostomy
- Risk for deficient fluid volume related to:
  - decreased intake
  - increased absorptive surface of distended bowel
  - nausea and vomiting
- Risk for infection of incision related to contamination from stools

Hypopituitarism

- Anxiety related to treatment regimen
- Risk for delayed development related to deficiency of anterior pituitary hormones
- Risk for disproportionate growth related to deficiency of anterior pituitary hormones

Hypospadias and epispadias

- Acute pain related to surgery
- Anxiety (child and parent) related to surgical procedure (urethroplasty)
- Risk for infection (urinary tract) related to placement of indwelling catheter
- Risk for injury related to dislodged urinary catheter or urinary catheter removal

Impetigo

- Deficient knowledge (treatment and prevention of recurrence of infection) related to new diagnosis
- Impaired skin integrity related to skin infection
- Risk for infection related to inadequate primary defenses

Intraventricular hemorrhage

- Deficient knowledge (infant's condition and potential for home care) related to the new injury
- Risk for injury related to fragility of the capillary beds in the cerebrum

Intussusception

- Acute pain related to bowel strangulation
- Anxiety (parent) related to surgery
- Nausea related to vomiting

Juvenile rheumatoid arthritis

- Chronic pain related to joint inflammation
- Disturbed body image related to the effects of the chronic illness and the disabling nature of the disease
- Impaired physical mobility related to joint inflammation
- Impaired skin integrity related to immobility
- Risk for imbalanced body temperature related to disease process

Kyphosis

- Disturbed body image related to altered physical appearance
- Readiness for enhanced management of therapeutic regimen related to readiness to follow treatment regimen
- Risk for situational low self-esteem related to altered physical appearance

Leukemia, acute

- Hopelessness related to illness
- Ineffective protection related to immunosuppression
- Risk for imbalanced body temperature related to infection
- Risk for infection related to altered primary and secondary defenses

Mononucleosis

- Fatigue related to weakness
- Interrupted family processes related to family member becoming temporary full-time caregiver
- Risk for imbalanced body temperature related to infection

Mumps

- Acute pain related to inflammation
- Fatigue related to infection
- Hyperthermia related to infection

Muscular dystrophy

- Caregiver role strain related to increased care needs
- Dressing/grooming, feeding self-care deficit related to muscle weakness and disability
- Impaired physical mobility related to muscle weakness
- Ineffective health maintenance related to inability to care for self

Myringotomy

- Anxiety (child and parent) related to the surgical procedure and perioperative events
- Deficient knowledge (home care procedures) related to new treatment
- Risk for injury (hemorrhage) related to surgery

Osteomyelitis

- Chronic pain related to inflammation and infection
- Compromised family coping related to prolonged hospital stay
- Imbalanced nutrition: Less than body requirements related to increased metabolic needs for wound healing
- Impaired physical mobility related to infection
- Impaired skin integrity related to infection
- Risk for infection related to wound contamination

Otitis media

- Acute pain related to inflammation of the middle ear
- Disturbed sensory perception (auditory) related to complications of otitis media
- Risk for infection related to impaired primary defenses

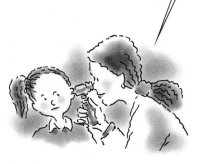

Some children with otitis media experience acute pain related to imflammation.

Pediculosis

- Impaired skin integrity related to itching and redness
- Situational low self-esteem related to lice
- Social isolation related to feelings of embarrassment due to diagnosis

Phenylketonuria

- Disturbed thought processes related to mental retardation
- Impaired skin integrity related to dry skin lesions
- Risk for delayed development related to accumulation of phenylalanine in blood

Protein-calorie malnutrition

- Imbalanced nutrition: Less than body requirements related to inability to ingest foods due to economic factors
- Ineffective protection related to malnutrition
- Risk for deficient fluid volume related to inability to ingest liquids due to economic factors

Pyloric stenosis

- Acute pain related to surgical incision
- Anxiety (parent) related to lack of understanding about the disease, diagnostic studies, and treatment
- Deficient fluid volume related to dehydration or shock (or both)
- Imbalanced nutrition: Less than body requirements related to frequent projectile vomiting
- Risk for infection related to surgery

Respiratory syncytial virus infection

- Imbalanced nutrition: Less than body requirements related to inability to ingest foods
- Ineffective breathing pattern related to decreased energy

• Risk for deficient fluid volume related to active loss and inflamed mucous membranes of the throat

Reye's syndrome

• Anxiety and fear (child) related to hospital stay
• Decreased intracranial adaptive capacity related to decreased cerebral perfusion
• Ineffective breathing pattern (with the potential for respiratory failure) related to cerebral edema
• Ineffective thermoregulation related to illness
• Ineffective tissue perfusion (cardiopulmonary, cerebral, renal) related to increased intracranial pressure (ICP)
• Ineffective tissue perfusion (cerebral) related to increased ICP and cerebral edema
• Risk for impaired parenting related to the child's hospital stay or lack of knowledge about the child's condition
• Risk for impaired skin integrity related to physical immobility
• Risk for injury (hypoglycemia) related to decreased calorie intake or possible metabolic dysfunction or both

Rheumatic fever and rheumatic heart disease

• Acute pain related to joint pain
• Decreased cardiac output related to carditis
• Hyperthermia related to infection

Roseola infantum

• Deficient knowledge (child's care needs and prognosis) related to new diagnosis
• Hyperthermia related to infection
• Impaired skin integrity related to skin rash

Rubella

• Deficient knowledge (child's care needs and prognosis) related to new diagnosis
• Hyperthermia related to infection
• Impaired skin integrity related to skin rash

Rubeola

• Fatigue related to disease
• Hyperthermia related to infection
• Impaired skin integrity related to pruritic rash

Scoliosis

• Acute pain related to curvature of spine
• Disturbed body image related to altered body shape
• Risk for impaired skin integrity related to brace

Sickle cell anemia

- Acute pain related to vascular occlusion and tissue hypoxia
- Deficient fluid volume related to decreased fluid intake and the kidneys' inability to concentrate urine
- Impaired gas exchange related to decreased oxygen-carrying capacity of blood
- Ineffective tissue perfusion (peripheral) related to blood vessel obstruction secondary to sickling of red blood cells

Spinal cord defects

- Deficient knowledge (spinal cord defects) related to lack of exposure to information
- Delayed growth and development related to spinal cord defect
- Disabled family coping related to increased caregiving demands on family with minimal social support

Tay-Sachs disease

- Delayed growth and development related to muscle weakness
- Disabled family coping related to family member with unexpressed feelings of anxiety
- Grieving related to death of child

Tonsillitis

- Acute pain related to throat swelling
- Hyperthermia related to infection
- Impaired swallowing related to swelling

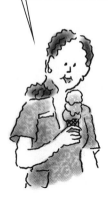

Tonsillitis can cause pain and difficulty swallowing. Luckily, ice cream slides right down!

Tracheoesophageal fistula

- Anxiety (parent) related to lack of knowledge about the disorder, diagnostic testing, and treatment
- Delayed growth and development related to the hospital stay and deprivation of normal parent-infant interactions and environmental stimulation
- Ineffective airway clearance related to aspiration of secretions or feedings or both
- Ineffective breathing pattern related to choking, coughing, and cyanosis during feeding

Tympanoplasty

- Anxiety (child and parent) related to surgical procedure and perioperative events
- Risk for injury (hemorrhage) related to surgery

Varicella

- Acute pain related to rash
- Impaired skin integrity related to itchy rash
- Interrupted family processes related to family member having to stay home from work to care for child

Psychiatric diagnoses

Just the facts

In this chapter, you'll learn:
♦ nursing diagnoses that correlate with common psychiatric medical diagnoses.

A look at psychiatric diagnoses

This chapter covers common psychiatric medical diagnoses. Each entry provides a list of a few of the major nursing diagnoses and related factors to be considered after your assessment of a patient with the particular medical diagnosis. Remember that the nursing diagnoses listed here represent the needs most commonly associated with the medical condition; your patient may have different needs.

Abusive disorders, sexual or physical

- Dysfunctional family processes related to violence
- Posttrauma syndrome related to:
  - interpersonal violence
  - physical neglect or abuse
  - sexual abuse or assault
- Risk for compromised human dignity related to abuse

Addictive disorders

Alcohol dependence

- Anxiety related to:
  - alcohol withdrawal
  - poor self-concept
  - real or perceived threats to physical safety
- Chronic low self-esteem related to:
  - coping difficulties
  - guilt
  - shame about alcohol abuse
  - unmet expectations
- Disturbed sensory perception (visual, auditory, tactile) related to acute alcohol withdrawal
- Dysfunctional family processes: Alcoholism related to role disruptions caused by the patient's alcohol-related disorder
- Imbalanced nutrition: Less than body requirements related to:
  - effects of chronic alcohol intake on digestive organs
  - interference of alcohol in absorption and metabolism of nutrients
  - poor dietary intake while consuming alcohol
- Insomnia related to alcohol abuse and decreased rapid eye movement sleep cycle
- Risk for injury related to:
  - alcohol withdrawal
  - depression
  - seizures
  - suicidal ideation
- Risk prone health behavior related to alcohol abuse

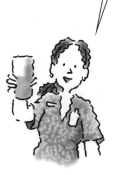

Alcohol dependence can lead to risk for injury related to withdrawal, depression, seizures, and suicidal ideation. Another reason to stay addicted to water. Cheers!

Hallucinogenic substance abuse

- Disturbed sensory perception (visual, auditory, kinesthetic, gustatory, tactile, olfactory) related to decreased cognitive function resulting from hallucinogen intake
- Disturbed thought processes related to:
  - hallucinogen abuse as evidenced by auditory or visual hallucinations
  - impaired memory
  - inattentiveness
  - problem-solving inabilities

- Insomnia related to hallucinogen abuse or intoxication as evidenced by verbal complaints of sleeping inability, nightmares, or interrupted sleep
- Risk for injury related to impaired judgment and disorientation
- Risk for injury related to poisoning by use of adulterated street drugs
- Risk prone health behavior related to substance abuse

Polysubstance abuse

- Chronic low self-esteem related to perceived failures and lack of positive feedback
- Disturbed sensory perception (visual, auditory, tactile) related to multiple psychoactive substance withdrawal
- Ineffective coping related to maladaptive reliance on alcohol and other drugs
- Powerlessness related to lack of control over psychoactive substance use

Stimulant abuse

- Decreased cardiac output related to stimulant use
- Deficient knowledge (risks of stimulant abuse) related to denial of need for information
- Disturbed sensory perception (visual, auditory, kinesthetic) related to sensory overload from stimulant use
- Fear related to altered thought processes
- Imbalanced nutrition: Less than body requirements related to placing greater importance on drug use than on eating
- Impaired social interaction related to isolation associated with drug use
- Ineffective health maintenance related to the effects of stimulant dependence on self-esteem
- Insomnia related to stimulant use
- Risk for imbalanced body temperature related to stimulant use
- Risk for impaired skin integrity related to changes in health maintenance
- Risk for other-directed violence related to:
  - difficulty processing and interpreting thoughts
  - sensory overload from stimulant use
- Risk prone health behavior related to substance abuse

Substance abuse (sedatives, opioids)

- Deficient knowledge (risks of substance abuse) related to inability to process or retain information while impaired and in denial
- Ineffective denial related to feelings of low self-esteem
- Risk for infection related to:
  - compromised immunity
  - high-risk behaviors
  - insufficient knowledge about disease
- Risk prone health behavior related to substance abuse

Adjustment disorder

- Complicated grieving related to:
  - inhibited grieving
  - multiple losses and bereavement processes
- Defensive coping related to:
  - inadequate support systems
  - personal vulnerability
  - unmet expectations
  - work overload
- Impaired social interaction related to decreased perception of appropriate social behavior
- Risk prone health behavior related to:
  - disability requiring lifestyle changes
  - impaired cognition
  - inadequate support systems
  - unresolved grieving

Anxiety disorder

- Anxiety related to:
  - stresses in home or work environments, close interpersonal relationships
  - threat to self-concept
  - unmet needs
- Chronic low self-esteem related to lack of positive feelings and difficulty concentrating
- Risk for imbalanced nutrition: Less than body requirements related to inability to ingest food due to psychological factors
- Social isolation related to panic state

Bipolar disorder

- Chronic low self-esteem related to depressive state and feelings of hopelessness, need to continue long-term medications
- Disturbed thought processes related to mood swings from mania to depression
- Impaired home maintenance related to difficulty concentrating and flight of ideas
- Sleep deprivation related to manic state

Delusional disorder

- Disturbed thought processes related to false beliefs that are based in reality
- Impaired social interaction related to delusional behavior
- Social isolation related to delusional behavior

Depression

- Chronic low self-esteem related to stress or loss
- Deficient diversional activity related to lack of interest
- Disturbed body image related to illness
- Imbalanced nutrition: More than or less than body requirements related to poor eating habits
- Ineffective coping related to obsessive negative thoughts and feelings
- Risk for caregiver role strain related to psychological needs of care receiver
- Risk for loneliness related to self-imposed social isolation
- Risk for self-directed violence related to self-help
- Social isolation related to inability to engage in satisfying personal relationships

Dissociative disorder

- Disturbed personal identity related to underdeveloped ego, threat to self-concept, or childhood abuse or trauma
- Ineffective coping related to a severe level of repressed anxiety
- Interrupted family processes related to shift in health status of family member

Eating disorders

- Deficient knowledge (nutrition and eating disorders) related to lack of interest in learning
- Disturbed body image related to misperceived physical appearance
- Imbalanced nutrition: Less than body requirements related to refusal to eat, purging activities, or excessive physical exercise
- Impaired social interaction related to withdrawal from peer group, fear of rejection, and preoccupation with eating behaviors or rituals
- Ineffective denial related to a lack of knowledge about real or potential dangers associated with eating disorders
- Interrupted family processes related to a perfectionistic, overprotective, or chaotic family system
- Risk for injury related to excessive exercise or potentially harmful behaviors

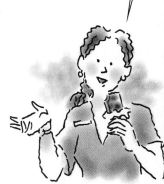

Preoccupation with eating behaviors or rituals can lead to impaired social interaction.

Gender identity disorder

- Anxiety related to conflict between desires and expected sex role behavior
- Disturbed personal identity related to conflict between anatomical sex and gender identity
- Ineffective sexuality pattern related to conflicts with sexual orientation
- Interrupted family processes related to family confusion and anxiety about gender of family member

Panic disorder

- Anxiety related to panic disorder
- Chronic low self-esteem related to repeated episodes of apprehension and fear
- Posttrauma syndrome related to perception of event or sudden loss

Personality disorder—Cluster A

- Impaired social interaction related to disorganized thinking, odd or eccentric behaviors, emotional coldness
- Ineffective coping related to:
  - inability to trust others
  - self-absorption
  - unusual perceptions and communication patterns
- Interrupted family processes related to shift in health status of family member

Personality disorder—Cluster B

- Impaired social interaction related to:
  - behaviors that produce hostility in others
  - inability to form healthy interpersonal relationships
  - low self-esteem
- Ineffective coping related to:
  - fear of abandonment
  - feelings of loneliness, emptiness, boredom
  - poor frustration tolerance
  - poor impulse control
- Risk for other-directed or self-directed violence related to dramatic, emotional, or erratic behavior or low self-esteem

Personality disorder—Cluster C

- Anxiety related to preoccupation
- Disturbed thought processes related to indecision or doubt over decisions
- Ineffective coping related to:
  - need to always be right and perfect
  - need to use rules and routines to maintain a secure environment
  - the inability to ask for help
  - verbal manipulation
- Interrupted family processes related to rigidity in functions, roles, and rules
- Powerlessness related to:
  - intellectualization or denial of feelings as a means to gain self-control
  - perfectionistic behavior that protects against inferiority feelings
- Sleep deprivation related to prolonged psychological discomfort
- Social isolation related to an inability to establish and maintain relationships

Phobias

- Disturbed personal identity related to inability to control fear
- Fear related to anxiety about an object or situation
- Ineffective coping related to persistent irrational fear

Posttraumatic stress disorder

- Hopelessness related to feelings of helplessness and loss of control
- Posttrauma syndrome related to traumatic event
- Powerlessness related to uncertainty about the future

Schizophrenia

- Anxiety related to disturbance in thought content
- Bathing/hygiene self-care deficit related to apathy and delusions
- Caregiver role strain related to chronic illness
- Disturbed thought processes related to genetic, biochemical, psychological, and sociocultural causes

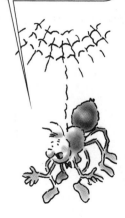

Persistent irrational fear can lead to ineffective coping. Stand back, folks. I'm about to drop in for a visit.

Sleep disorder

- Anxiety related to inability to sleep
- Insomnia related to:
  - external factors, such as hospital routines, environmental noise, and changing work shifts
  - medical illness
  - pain
  - psychological stress
- Interrupted family processes related to family member not being able to fulfill role requirements because of lack of sleep

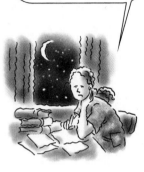

Patients with sleep disorders can experience anxiety related inability to sleep. At this point, even the sheep have gone to sleep.

Somatoform and factitious disorders

- Bathing/hygiene, dressing/grooming self-care deficit related to:
  - activity intolerance
  - neuromuscular or musculoskeletal impairment
  - pain or discomfort
  - perceptual or cognitive impairment
- Caregiver role strain related to unpredictable illness and conflict with care receiver
- Chronic pain related to unmet dependency needs or repressed anxiety as demonstrated by verbal complaints with no pathophysiologic validation
- Deficient knowledge (healthful social interactions) related to:
  - denial
  - intense repressed anxiety level
  - lack of interest in learning
  - preoccupation with self and pain
- Disabled family coping related to struggle for control and power
- Disturbed body image related to low self-esteem evidenced by preoccupation with real or imagined altered body structure or function
- Ineffective coping related to:
  - extreme need for approval and acceptance
  - inability to manage emotional conflict
  - low self-esteem
  - unmet dependency needs
- Social isolation related to physical symptoms or disability

Vicarious traumatization

- Insomnia related to recurrent nightmares or dreams of personal death and fear of their recurrence
- Posttrauma syndrome related to the subjective experience of single or multiple traumatic events through repeated exposure to trauma victims (vicarious traumatization)
- Powerlessness related to:
  - inadequate problem-solving and coping skills
  - overwhelming anxiety

Appendices and index

NANDA-I nursing diagnoses by domain   272

Selected references   274

Index   275

NANDA-I nursing diagnoses by domain

This list presents the 2007-2008 NANDA International (NANDA-I)
taxonomy II according to their domains.

Domain: Health promotion

- Effective therapeutic regimen management
- Health-seeking behaviors (specify)
- Impaired home maintenance
- Ineffective community therapeutic regimen management
- Ineffective family therapeutic regimen management
- Ineffective health maintenance
- Ineffective therapeutic regimen management
- Readiness for enhanced immunization status
- Readiness for enhanced nutrition
- Readiness for enhanced therapeutic regimen management

Domain: Nutrition

- Deficient fluid volume
- Excess fluid volume
- Imbalanced nutrition: Less than body requirements
- Imbalanced nutrition: More than body requirements
- Impaired swallowing
- Ineffective infant feeding pattern
- Readiness for enhanced fluid balance
- Risk for deficient fluid volume
- Risk for imbalanced fluid volume
- Risk for imbalanced nutrition: More than body requirements
- Risk for impaired liver function
- Risk for unstable blood glucose level

Domain: Elimination/Exchange

- Bowel incontinence
- Constipation
- Diarrhea
- Functional urinary incontinence
- Impaired gas exchange
- Impaired urinary elimination
- Overflow urinary incontinence
- Perceived constipation
- Readiness for enhanced urinary elimination
- Reflex urinary incontinence
- Risk for constipation
- Risk for urge urinary incontinence
- Stress urinary incontinence
- Total urinary incontinence
- Urge urinary incontinence
- Urinary retention

Domain: Activity/Rest

- Activity intolerance
- Bathing/hygiene self-care deficit
- Decreased cardiac output
- Deficient diversional activity
- Delayed surgical recovery
- Dressing/grooming self-care deficit
- Dysfunctional ventilatory weaning response

- Energy field disturbance
- Fatigue
- Feeding self-care deficit
- Impaired bed mobility
- Impaired physical mobility
- Impaired spontaneous ventilation
- Impaired transfer ability
- Impaired walking
- Impaired wheelchair mobility
- Ineffective breathing pattern
- Ineffective tissue perfusion (specify type: renal, cerebral, cardiopulmonary, gastrointestinal, peripheral)
- Insomnia
- Readiness for enhance self-care
- Readiness for enhanced sleep
- Risk for activity intolerance
- Risk for disuse syndrome
- Sedentary lifestyle
- Sleep deprivation
- Toileting self-care deficit

Domain: Perception/Cognition

- Acute confusion
- Chronic confusion
- Deficient knowledge (specify)
- Disturbed sensory perception (specify: visual, auditory, kinesthetic, gustatory, tactile)
- Disturbed thought processes
- Impaired environmental interpretation syndrome
- Impaired memory
- Impaired verbal communication
- Readiness for enhanced communication
- Readiness for enhanced decision making
- Readiness for enhanced knowledge (specify)
- Risk for acute confusion
- Unilateral neglect
- Wandering

Domain: Self-perception

- Chronic low self-esteem
- Disturbed body image
- Disturbed personal identity
- Hopelessness
- Powerlessness
- Readiness for enhanced power
- Risk for compromised human dignity
- Readiness for enhanced hope
- Readiness for enhanced self-concept
- Risk for loneliness
- Risk for powerlessness
- Risk for situational low self-esteem
- Situational low self-esteem

Domain: Role relationships

- Caregiver role strain
- Dysfunctional family processes: Alcoholism
- Effective breast-feeding
- Impaired parenting
- Impaired social interaction
- Ineffective breast-feeding
- Ineffective role performance
- Interrupted breast-feeding
- Interrupted family processes
- Parental role conflict
- Readiness for enhanced family processes
- Readiness for enhanced parenting
- Risk for caregiver role strain
- Risk for impaired parent/infant/child attachment
- Risk for impaired parenting

Domain: Sexuality

- Ineffective sexuality pattern
- Sexual dysfunction

Domain: Coping/Stress tolerance

- Anxiety
- Autonomic dysreflexia
- Chronic sorrow
- Complicated grieving
- Compromised family coping
- Death anxiety
- Decreased intracranial adaptive capacity
- Defensive coping
- Disabled family coping
- Disorganized infant behavior
- Fear
- Grieving
- Ineffective community coping
- Ineffective coping
- Ineffective denial
- Post-trauma syndrome
- Rape-trauma syndrome
- Rape-trauma syndrome: Compound reaction
- Rape-trauma syndrome: Silent reaction
- Readiness for enhanced community coping
- Readiness for enhanced coping (individual)
- Readiness for enhanced family coping
- Readiness for enhanced organized infant behavior
- Relocation stress syndrome
- Risk for autonomic dysreflexia
- Risk for complicated grieving
- Risk for disorganized infant behavior
- Risk for post-trauma syndrome
- Risk for relocation stress syndrome
- Risk-prone health behavior
- Stress overload

Domain: Life principles

- Decisional conflict (specify)
- Impaired religiosity
- Moral distress

- Noncompliance (specify)
- Readiness for enhanced decision making
- Readiness for enhanced religiosity
- Readiness for enhanced spiritual well-being
- Readiness for enhanced hope
- Risk for impaired religiosity
- Risk for spiritual distress
- Spiritual distress

Domain: Safety/Protection

- Contamination
- Hyperthermia
- Hypothermia
- Impaired dentition
- Impaired oral mucous membrane
- Impaired skin integrity
- Impaired tissue integrity
- Ineffective airway clearance
- Ineffective protection
- Ineffective thermoregulation
- Latex allergy response
- Readiness for enhanced immunization status
- Risk for aspiration
- Risk for contamination
- Risk for falls
- Risk for imbalanced body temperature
- Risk for impaired skin integrity
- Risk for infection
- Risk for injury
- Risk for latex allergy response
- Risk for other-directed violence
- Risk for perioperative positioning injury
- Risk for peripheral neurovascular dysfunction
- Risk for poisoning
- Risk for self-directed violence
- Risk for self-mutilation
- Risk for sudden infant death syndrome
- Risk for suffocation
- Risk for suicide
- Risk for trauma
- Self-mutilation

Domain: Comfort

- Acute pain
- Chronic pain
- Nausea
- Readiness for enhanced comfort
- Social isolation

Domain: Growth/Development

- Adult failure to thrive
- Delayed growth and development
- Risk for delayed development
- Risk for disproportionate growth

© NANDA International. (2007). *NANDA-I Nursing Diagnoses: Definitions & Classifications 2007-2008*. Philadelphia: NANDA International. Reprinted with permission.

Selected references

Carpenito-Moyet, L.J. *Nursing Care Plans & Documentation: Nursing Diagnosis and Collaborative Problems*, 4th ed. Philadelphia: Lippincott Williams & Wilkins, 2004.

Carpenito-Moyet, L.J. *Understanding the Nursing Process: Concept Mapping and Care Planning for Students.* Philadelphia: Lippincott Williams & Wilkins, 2007.

Ignatavicius, D., and Workman, M.L. *Medical-Surgical Nursing: Critical Thinking for Collaborative Care*, 5th ed. Philadelphia: W.B. Saunders Co., 2006.

Johnson, M., et al. *NANDA, NOC, and NIC Linkages*, 2nd ed. Philadelphia: Mosby, 2006.

Klossner, N.J. *Introductory Maternity Nursing.* Philadelphia: Lippincott Williams & Wilkins, 2006.

McCloskey-Dochterman, J., and Bulechek, G., eds. *Nursing Interventions Classification (NIC)*, 4th ed. St. Louis: Mosby, 2004.

Moorehead, S., et al., eds. *Iowa Outcomes Project: Nursing Outcomes Classification (NOC)*, 3rd ed. St. Louis: Mosby, 2004.

Nursing Diagnoses: Definitions & Classifications 2007-2008. Philadelphia: NANDA International, 2007.

Nursing Student Success Made Incredibly Easy. Philadelphia: Lippincott Williams & Wilkins, 2005.

Shives, L. *Concepts of Psychiatric-Mental Health Nursing*, 7th ed. Philadelphia: Lippincott Williams & Wilkins, 2007.

Smeltzer, S. *Brunner and Suddarth's Textbook of Medical-Surgical Nursing*, 11th ed. Philadelphia: Lippincott Williams & Wilkins, 2007.

Sparks-Ralph, S., and Taylor, C. *Sparks and Taylor's Nursing Diagnosis Reference Manual*, 6th ed. Philadelphia: Lippincott Williams & Wilkins, 2005.

Wong, D., et al. *Maternal Child Nursing Care*, 3rd ed. Philadelphia: Mosby, 2006.

Index

A

Abuse, asking about, in nursing history, 28
Activities of daily living, nursing history and, 27
Activity and exercise pattern, assessing, 40
Actual diagnosis, 64-65
Acute care hospital unit, care plan in, 168-170
Administration route, incorrect,
    avoiding, 130
Advanced practice nurse as health care team
    member, 136
Air bubbles in pump tubing, avoiding, 130
Alternative clinical requirements, nursing
    shortage and, 122
Alternative clinical settings, nursing shortage
    and, 122
American Nurses Association
  NANDA International and, 14
  nursing process and, 6
Assessment
  complete, 24
    components of, 24-34, 38-39
  critical thinking and, 12
  of current patient situation, 123-124, 125-127i,
    127-128
  data collection and, 23
  focused, 24
  initial, Joint Commission standards for, 43
  integrating, into caregiving tasks, 51-52
  as nursing process step, 8, 23-56
Auscultation as examination technique, 32
Autonomy versus shame and doubt developmen-
    tal stage, 49

B

Bedside shift report, 124
Behavior as element in outcome statement,
    89-90, 90i
Biographic data, nursing history and, 26

C

Calculation errors, avoiding, 130
Caregiving tasks, integrating assessment into,
    51-52

Care plan. *See also* Care planning.
  in acute care hospital unit, 168-170
  changing, 11, 154-156, 155i
  collaborative care and, 75-77
  components of, 87-88
  computerized, 167-168
  creating, 174-175
  documenting, 10
  evaluating, 153
  in extended-care facilities, 170-171
  flexibility of, 11
  in hospice setting, 174
  implementing, 119-140
  individually developed, 163-165, 164i
  purpose of, 3
  reassessment of, 152-153
  as required part of patient's record, 159-161
  in same-day surgery unit, 170
  sample
    for maternal-neonatal care, 177-178t
    for pediatric care, 183t
    for psychiatric care, 180-181t
  standardized, 165, 166i, 167
  traditional, 163-165, 164i
  updating, 154-156, 155i
  versus concept map, 18t
Care planning. *See also* Care plan.
  in health care setting, 161
  nursing process and, 3-4, 6
  patient input in, 4, 94-95, 96
  students' role in, 161-162
Clinical instructors, level of responsibility and, 121
Clinical nurse specialist as health care team
    member, 136
Clinical partnerships, nursing shortage and, 122
Clinical preceptorships, nursing shortage and, 122
Clinical site staff, level of responsibility
    and, 121, 162
Cognition and perception, assessing, 42
Collaborative care, 75-77
Collaborative interventions, 105, 106i
Complete assessment, 24
  components of, 24-24, 38-39

i refers to an illustration; t refers to a table.

Concept map, 17. *See also* Concept mapping.
  creating, 18-19
    based on assessment data, 52-54, 55i, 56
    guidelines for, 19
  creating nursing diagnoses from, 67, 68i, 69
  sample
    for maternal-neonatal care, 176i
    for pediatric care, 182i
    for psychiatric care, 179i
  uses for, 19
Concept mapping. *See also* Concept map.
  advantages of, 17
  disadvantages of, 17-18
  versus nursing care plans, 18t
Conditions as element in outcome statement, 90i,
      91-92
Consultant specialty physician as health
      care team member, 136
Coping and stress management pattern,
      assessing, 42
Critical observation as examination technique, 32
Critical pathway, 170, 172-173i
Critical thinking, 11-13
  as essential skill, 13
  hallmarks of, 12-13
  nursing process and, 12-13
Cultural influences, nursing history and, 29-30
Current complaints, nursing history and, 26
Current patient situation, assessment of, as imple-
      mentation step, 123-124, 125-127i, 127-128

D
Data collection
  assessment and, 23
  organization and, 39-40, 41i, 42-43, 44-47i, 48
Developmental stages
  autonomy versus shame and doubt, 49
  generativity versus self-absorption, 50-51
  identity versus role confusion, 50
  industry versus inferiority, 50
  initiative versus guilt, 50
  integrity versus despair, 51
  intimacy versus isolation, 50
  trust versus mistrust, 49
Diagnostic statement, 62. *See also* Nursing diag-
      nosis.
  writing, 70-73, 75-77
Diagnostic testing data, assessment and, 33
Differential diagnosis, 31

Discharge planner as health care team
      member, 136
Documentation
  of care plan, 10
  of changes in patient's condition, 150
  patient-centered, 136
Documentation formats, 137-140, 139i, 140i
Domains
  in NANDA International-approved nursing
      diagnoses, 70, 71, 102, 109
  in Nursing Interventions Classification
      system, 109
  in Nursing Outcomes Classification system,
      98-99, 102, 109
Drug information
  collecting, 35-36t
  reliable resources for, 37-38
Drug orders, 130
Drug preparation and administration, 130

E
Electronic health record, 167-168
Electronic shift report, 125-127i
Elimination pattern, assessing, 40
Erikson's stages of development, 49-51
Etiology as nursing diagnosis part, 63
Evaluation
  of care plan, 153
  critical thinking and, 12
  Likert scales as tool for, 99, 100
  of long-term goals, 151-152
  as nursing process step, 11, 143
  reassessment and, 144-150
  of short-term goals, 151
  value of, 143-144
Evaluation statements, writing, 150-152
Evidence-based practice, 112-113
Extended-care facility
  care plan in, 170-171
  RN Assessment Coordinator in, 171

F
Family history, nursing history and, 30
Five rights of drug administration, 129, 131
Focused assessment, 24
Focus factor, patient interactions and, 12
Follow-up assessment data, comparing, with prior,
      144-146
Food and Drug Administration, 37

i refers to an illustration; t refers to a table.

Functional levels, assigning codes to, 41i. *See also* Gordon's functional health patterns.

G

General survey of patient, 31-32
Generativity versus self-absorption as developmental stage, 50-51
Gordon's functional health patterns, 39-43
    assigning codes to levels of, 41i
    categories included in, 39-40, 42-43
    NANDA International Taxonomy II and, 70
Growth and development stages, 48-51

H

Health perception and management pattern, assessing, 40
Herbal products, information resources for, 37, 38
Hospice
    care plan in, 174
    interdisciplinary team in, 136

I

Identity versus role confusion as developmental stage, 50
Implementation
    assessment of current situation and, 123-124, 125-127i, 127-128
    basic steps in, 129, 131
    as nursing process step, 11, 119-120
Independent interventions, 104-105, 106i
Industry versus inferiority developmental stage, 50
Information sources, evaluating, 112-113
Initiative versus guilt developmental stage, 50
Inspection as examination technique, 32
Integrated database format, 43, 44-47i
Integrating nursing care, 131-132, 135
Integrity versus despair as developmental stage, 51
Interdependent interventions, 105, 106i
Interdisciplinary team
    care planning and, 161
    working with, 135-137
Interventions
    care plan and, 10
    correlating, with patient outcomes, 96
    documenting, 137-140
    evaluating, 147, 148i, 149-150
    keeping track of, 147
    standardized classification system for, 15, 16

Interventions *(continued)*
    types of, 104-105, 106i
    using Nursing Interventions Classification to write, 109-111, 110i
    writing, 105, 107-108
Intimacy versus isolation as developmental stage, 50

JK

Joint Commission
    as authority on practice standards, 160
    standards of, for initial assessments, 43
Joint student experiences, nursing shortage and, 122

L

Label as nursing diagnosis part, 63
Language barrier, overcoming, 30
Levels of responsibility, 120-121, 123
Likert scales as evaluation tool, 99, 101
Long-term goals, evaluating, 151-152

M

Maslow's hierarchy of needs, 83i
Maternal-neonatal diagnoses, 245-250
Measure as element in outcome statement, 90i, 91
Medical diagnoses versus nursing diagnoses, 9, 77, 79-80t
Medical diagnosis, reviewing, 38-39
Medical procedure data, reviewing, 34, 38
Medical-surgical diagnoses, 191-244
Medication use, current, reviewing, 34
Mind map. *See* Concept map.
Modifications to care plan, 154-156, 155i
Multidisciplinary admission form, 44-47i

N

NANDA International, 14, 70. *See also* NANDA International-approved diagnoses.
    submitting new diagnoses to, 72i
NANDA International-approved diagnoses, 14, 16. *See also* NANDA International.
    choosing, 78i
    definition of, 61-62
    diagnostic statements and, 70-73, 75-77
    by domain, 272-273
    domains in, 70, 71
    Taxonomy II for, 70
    levels of, 70, 71

i refers to an illustration; t refers to a table.

National Patient Safety Goals, 128
North American Nursing Diagnosis Association.
        See NANDA International.
Nurse-manager as health care team member, 136
Nurse practitioner as health care team
        member, 136
Nurses as resources, 129
\Nursing diagnosis
    actual versus risk for, 8
    classifications system for, 14
    collaborative care and, 75-77
    components of, 9-10
    creating, from concept map, 67, 68i, 69
    critical thinking and, 12
    developing a problem list for, 69, 69i
    do's and don'ts of writing, 74-75
    formulating, 62
    as nursing process step, 8, 61-83
    parts of, 62-63, 64
    prioritizing, 82-83
        Maslow's pyramid and, 83i
    types of, 63-66
    validating, 80, 81i, 82
    versus medical diagnoses, 9, 77, 79-80t
Nursing diagnoses by medical diagnosis, 189-270
    maternal-neonatal diagnoses, 245-250
    medical-surgical diagnoses, 191-244
    pediatric diagnoses, 251-262
    psychiatric diagnoses, 263-270
Nursing history, 25-30
Nursing Interventions Classification system, 15, 16,
        108-109
    domains in, 108-109
    using, to write interventions, 109, 110i, 111
Nursing Outcomes Classification system, 15, 16,
        95-96, 98-102
    anatomy of outcome in, 100i
    categories in, 98-99
    definition of outcome in, 98
    role of Likert scales in, 99, 101
    using, to write expected outcomes, 101-102,
        103-104i
Nursing process, 3-4
    advantages of, 4-5
    basis for, 5
    critical thinking and, 11-13
    initial definition of, 6
    postgraduation use of, 13-14
    reassessment throughout, 145t

Nursing process, *(continued)*
    steps in, 5-6, 8-11
        interrelationship of, 6, 7i, 8
Nursing shortage, 122
Nursing student, level of responsibility and, 120,
        121, 161-162
Nutrition and metabolism pattern,
        assessing, 40

O
Objective data, 25
Occupational therapist as health care team
        member, 136
Off-label drug uses, 37
Outcome-oriented documentation, 136
Outcomes, expected
    achieving, 149-150
    adapting, to specific circumstances, 94, 95i
    care plan and, 10
    correlating, with specific interventions, 96
    critical thinking and, 13
    evaluating, 147, 148i
    identifying, 88-95
    standardized classification system for, 15
    using Nursing Outcomes Classification to write,
        101-102
Outcome statement, 89
    parts of, 89-92, 90i
    patient input in, 94-95, 96
    specificity and conciseness in, 93-94, 100i
    writing, 92-95, 97-98
Over-the-counter drugs, information resources
        for, 37, 38

PQ
Palliative care, interdisciplinary team in, 136
Palpation as examination technique, 32
Past medical history, nursing history and, 26-27
Pastoral care specialist as health care team
        member, 136
Patient assessment data, comparing prior, with
        follow-up, 144-146
Patient-centered documentation, 136
Patient compliance, improving, 96
Patient goals, 10
    long-term, 92
        documenting, 93
        evaluating, 151-152
    short-term, 92
        evaluating, 151

i refers to an illustration; t refers to a table.

Patient outcomes. *See* Outcomes, expected.
Patient safety goals, 128
Patient's chart as data source, 33
Pediatric diagnoses, 251-262
Percussion as examination technique, 32
Pharmacist as health care team member, 136
Physical examination, 31-32
  general survey and, 31-32
  goals of, 31
  techniques used in, 32
Physical therapist as health care team
    member, 136
Physician as health care team member, 136
Physician's assistant as health care team
    member, 136
Planning as nursing process step, 10
Plan of care. *See* Care plan.
Prescription drugs, information resources
    for, 37-38
Primary nurse as health care team
    member, 136
Prioritizing nursing diagnoses, 82-83
  Maslow's pyramid and, 83i
Problem-intervention-evaluation documentation
    system, 138, 139i
Problem list, developing, 69, 69i
Problem solving as basis for nursing
    process, 5
Psychiatric diagnoses, 263-270

R
Reassessment
  of care plan, 152-153
  nursing process and, 144, 145t
  of patient, 144-150
Registered dietitian as health care team
    member, 136
Respiratory therapist as health care team
    member, 136
Risk diagnosis, 65
RN Assessment Coordinator in extended-care
    facility, 171
Roles and relationships, assessing, 42

S
Safe drug administration guidelines, 130
Same-day surgery unit, care plan in, 170
Self-perception and self-concept,
    assessing, 42

Sexuality and reproduction pattern,
    assessing, 42
Shift report
  bedside, 124
  electronic, 125-127i
Short-term goals, evaluating, 151
Signs and symptoms as nursing diagnosis part, 63
Sleep and rest pattern, assessing, 42
SOAP documentation format, 138-140, 140i
Social worker as health care team
    member, 136
Socioeconomic factors, nursing history and, 29
Specialty database formats, 43, 48
Spiritual influences, nursing history and, 29, 30
Staff nurse, level of responsibility and, 121
Standardized care plans, 165, 166i, 167
  advantages of, 167
  disadvantage of, 167
STOP acronym, 54
Stressors, nursing history and, 27, 28
Subjective data, 25
Support systems, nursing history and, 27-28
Syndrome diagnosis, 65-66

TU
Time frame as element in outcome statement, 90i,
    92
Traditional care plan, 163-165, 164i
  advantages of, 163-164
  basic form for, 163, 164i
  disadvantage of, 165
Trust versus mistrust developmental stage, 49

V
Validating nursing diagnoses, 80, 81i, 82
Values and beliefs, assessing, 43

WXYZ
Wellness diagnosis, 66

i refers to an illustration; t refers to a table.

Ready to start writing a care plan?

Well, we've made it easier by including *Nursing Care Planning Made Incredibly Easy Care Planner*, a CD-ROM with more than 150 customizable care plans from every nursing specialty. Just install the program, choose a care plan, and you're ready to edit the care plan using the features available in your word processing program. Remember to save your changes!

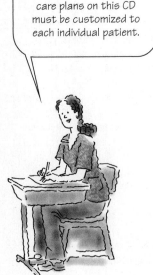

Remember that the care plans on this CD must be customized to each individual patient.

Technical stuff

To operate the *Nursing Care Planning Made Incredibly Easy Care Planner* CD-ROM, we recommend that you have the following minimum system requirements:
- Windows XP Home Edition
- Microsoft Word
- Pentium 4
- 512 MB RAM
- 40 MB of free hard-disk space
- SVGA monitor with high color (16-bit); display area set to 800 × 600
- CD-ROM drive.

Getting started

- Start Windows.
- Place the CD in your CD-ROM drive. After a few moments, the install process will automatically begin. *Note:* If the install process doesn't automatically begin, click the Start menu and select Run. Type *D:\setup.exe* (where *D:* is the letter of your CD-ROM drive) and then click OK.
- Follow the on-screen instructions for the installation type you want.

It's that easy!

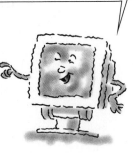

For technical support, call toll-free 1-800-638-3030, Monday through Friday, 8:30 a.m. to 5 p.m. Eastern Time. Or, e-mail us at wkhealth-support@wolterskluwer.com.